Inviting Everyone:
Healing Healthcare through
Positive Deviance

Arvind Singhal
Prucia Buscell
Curt Lindberg

PlexusPress
Bordentown, New Jersey

For permissions contact: info@plexusinstitute.org

PlexusPress
www.PlexusInstitute.org

Design by David Hutchens, Iconoclast Communications

ISBN: 1453731644

Contents

This book is dedicated to

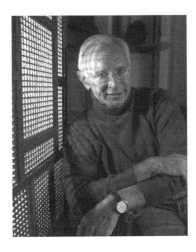

Jerry Sternin
(1938-2008)

who believed in the wisdom of all people, and helped unleash it to save and to improve the lives of millions around the world.

Those who knew Jerry Sternin have no doubt heard him recount the story of Nasirudin, the Sufi mystic who, depending on the lesson to be emphasized, took on various guises.

In one story, Nasirudin appears as a smuggler who, riding a donkey, arrives at the customs checkpoint each evening. The custom inspector, intent on catching Nasirudin in an act of wrongdoing, would feverishly search the contents of the hung baskets, finding nothing but straw. Years go by, the search routine continues, and Nasirudin grows richer and richer. One day Nasirudin retires from smuggling, and happens to meet the customs inspector, now also retired.

"Tell me, Nasirudin," pleads his former adversary, "now that you have nothing to hide, and I have nothing to find, what was it that you were smuggling all those years?"

Nasirudin replies, "Donkeys, of course!"

Jerry would tell this story to make the following point: too often the reality, the answer, the truth, lies right in front of our eyes, but we do not see it. Such is especially true of experts who are trained to "look in baskets" akin to the customs inspector. Such affliction of experts can also be termed "occupational psychosis" or "trained incapacity." Positive Deviance is an approach based on the premise that the solutions to intractable problems are right there, with the community members, staring us in the face. Use of the PD process helps to make these invisible solutions visible to everyone.

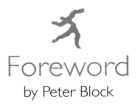

Foreword
by Peter Block

The Positive Deviance (PD) movement is changing the landscape of how we achieve transformation and change in systems. This book is a big step forward in defining this new landscape. And what fun to see it take a foothold in the big conversation about health care reform. PD is much more radical than even its practitioners imagine. Radical in the best sense, it is joining a new field of inquiry, which might be called communal transformation.

We all have a long tradition of thinking about individual transformation, but the question of how collectives or social systems are transformed by design is still open for discovery. We are familiar with how social systems can be disrupted by forces like technology, or shifts in markets, or political upheaval, but how to reform a social system growing out of the explicit intention of its own members is still cluttered with conventional practices that struggle to fulfill what they were designed to do.

Most of our efforts at changing organizational or community cultures have not succeeded. This is where I think PD has something special and fresh to offer. Even the progressive conventional thinking on how to change organizational culture and behavior is still based on a fourfold worldview:

1. *We believe that improvement comes from more consistency and control.* When something goes wrong and needs changing, like MRSA, our first instinct is to prescribe more oversight, closer watching, clearer consequences, and more predictability. Even the very successful TPS or Toyota system mentioned in the book makes a heavy bet on consistency and eliminating exceptions. As one of the examples you will read about in the book, total quality can create order, and there is the story and image of how, through a quality process, a utility room became more efficient and satisfying to its users. Who would not want to walk into a utility room where everything is labeled and in order? That is a good metaphor for what today's total quality movement tries to achieve in not only the order of a room but in the order of social systems. More order is not what is transformative.

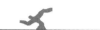

There is no evidence that high controls lead to either high performance or better quality.

We, however, are a bit stuck on order and confuse it with transformation. Eliminating exceptions and waste reduction are good things, but not the main point. Methods for consistency and control are a good fit with health care since you might have noticed that there are few industries more filled with oversight and regulation than health care.

This book is on a very different path than more control and order. That is what is exciting here. It confronts us with our love affair with more controls, and is clear eyed that more control does not prove to be effective. There is no evidence that high controls lead to either high performance or better quality. What control gives us is defensibility. In a punitive, highly litigious culture, a culture that cares more about who is to blame than what we can learn, more oversight keeps us out of trouble; it does not produce more health.

This is why the health care reform conversation is not changing anything; it is all about cost and controls. There is no reform in this. No shift in thinking. It is only about trying harder at what is not working so well now.

2. *We believe that data is persuasive, especially when gathered by expert, objective third parties.* There is a great quote in Chapter 6 of this book that declares that "…action can proceed in parallel with the elusive quest for unequivocal data accuracy: Physicians will make changes if they are presented with applicable data that demonstrates the need for change. Physicians want perfection, have high standards and expect everyone to function at a high level. Data helps drive their decisions." Oh, that this were true. This is not to question the learning capacities of physicians. It is just that there is a long history of ineffective change efforts that were driven by burning platforms, long data collection, close analysis, and reasoned need for change.

The grip and power of social systems to stay in place is hard to unfreeze with more data.

We need only to look at one common feature of traditional change management: the first step is to identify "the gap"—that is, data about the distance between where things stand now and where we want to be in the future. Even when we carefully research this gap, and find tight measures of where we are now and where we want to be, the reasoned, persuasive argument for the need for change is rarely compelling. Interesting? Always. But this rarely results in real social inventions. The grip and power of social systems to stay in place is hard to unfreeze with more data. Otherwise innovations would not take so long to find widespread use.

The book offers an example of this in the story of Dr. Semmelweis. He had evidence that hand washing saved lives. He was inspired, committed, had data on his side. But the evidence was contrary to the conventional wisdom, and nothing shifted. He ended his life questioning what he knew to be true. We had to wait until the germ was discovered to realize what he knew to be true. His story exemplifies the difficulty of acting on what we know.

Measurement and assessment play an important role in the Positive Deviant way of solving the unsolvable. But in my view, it is the dispersed ways of having core workers collect data, share the data and invent clever ways of communicating the data that is unique here.

Very different from the conventional strategies of finding the right answer, disseminating it, launching education efforts and taking ideas to scale.

3. *We believe that strong leadership and support from the top is essential to transformation.* Early in every story of attempted transformation,

our attention goes to the leader and how they enabled the effort. Or if the effort failed, we first look at the lack of senior leadership to explain what happened. That is why the stories in this book are important, because in almost every instance people at the top facilitated or allowed the effort, but they were not the role models or initiators or champions. This came from those in the middle. The leaders, at best, learned a new way of leading. They learned to listen and support. The success of these efforts in no way can be placed at the feet of top management. If, in reading these stories, you stay focused on the role of those at the top, the power of the story is passing you by.

The stories in this book are important, because in almost every instance people at the top allowed the effort, but they were not the role models or champions.

The profound potential for large-scale communal reform in these stories is suggested by the fact that PD is making a difference in an industry where there exists a strong tradition and commitment to patriarchy, in health care systems that have become the leading paragon of the belief in clear class divisions, the power of the high-status person in the system, and vivid distinctions of who in the room is authorized to speak with authority.

4. *We think that if we can identify a problem, we can solve it.* We love problem solving. We are drawn to deficiencies. It is the engineer in each of us that dominates most conversations. If you want to raise money, you have to be able to point to a need and name what is missing or the cause of suffering. This was true in the Sternins' experience and the story of Positive Deviance up to this point.

The reality is that more problem solving does not create an alternative future. It is not the methodology of transformation. Just because we can measure and quantify the world, it does not mean it will change. Something more powerful needs to be confronted.

Invisible and Close at Hand

The Positive Deviance work is not fundamentally dependent on these four premises. Nor does it ignore or argue against the value of control and consistency, or the need for accurate data, or the help that progressive leadership can provide, or the importance of problem solving. There is no argument there. These are all good things. However, you can see in the PD stories that prior strategies based on the dominant cultural beliefs were not decisive when communal transformation, or a shift in a social system, is what was required.

All change efforts failed at exactly the moment in which we now found ourselves —the moment at which the solution was discovered.

This is a key point. Social systems are human systems. They are complex systems, as mentioned in the book. Which means that they cannot be reasoned, persuaded, driven, engineered, or implemented into an alternative way of functioning. They have to be invited, enticed, seduced, engaged into participating in what could be called a self-inflicted wound. Real change in human systems has to be bought, it cannot be sold. The easy term for this is self-organizing or self-managing change.

This is what the Sternins figured out. Wherever they went, they knew that having the traditional change management and development strategies would not make the difference. They knew that having the right answer, teaching the right answer, leaning on leaders, and relying on reason-based approaches were of little value. There is a quote from their own book (*The Power of Positive Deviance: How Unlikely Innovators Solve the World's Toughest Problems*) that is telling. After finding examples of the positive deviants, the Sternins realized that having the answer was the point where most change efforts fail. "All [failures] had occurred exactly at the moment in which we now found ourselves—the moment at which the solution (aka the 'truth') is discovered. The next, almost reflexive step was to go out and spread the word: teach people, tell them, educate them...we realized that [failures] occurred because we were acting as though once people 'know' something it results in them 'doing' something."

So the stories in the book really just begin at the point when the initiators had data on their side. They had proof that innovative practices in hand washing and protection would save lives and suffering. Now what do they do, other than launch a selling effort, find champions, get the top on their side, do the best practices routine, find some catchy acronym or slogan? This is where the best ones got smart. And got radical.

Here is what they did that was unique and what I would bet on any day to loosen and touch a social system and produce something sustainable and scalable:

1. *They looked for signs of health.* Counter cultural in a disease oriented "health" industry. But they did it. They resisted the gap analysis. They didn't look to changing the reward system. Or starting trainings. Or ranking people on their performance. Not doing the wrong thing counts.

2. *They decided to listen.* They organized a process of profound listening. Brought groups together to discover what is working. And when they got some answers, they brought more groups together to listen some more. Most improvement efforts are about profound speaking. And if the message is not working, turn up the volume. PD is only about the listening.

3. *They chose positive intent with each person they contacted.* They acted on faith, rather than cynicism. They did not talk about resistance to change; they caught people at their best. They held the wisdom of citizens at every level in esteem. They authorized people on the margin and lower levels to speak. Core workers spoke and physicians listened. If this did not happen, nothing would have changed. Some of the stories in the book call this "better communication and engagement." That expression sterilizes what was going on. It misses the radical nature of this approach. This was a revolution in the communal belief about whose voice matters.

4. *In each story, top leadership was tolerant and often played a supportive but relatively minor role.* Not to discount their place or say the leaders did not matter, because of course they do. It is just that this ap-

proach simply avoids the deference to position that is so common in most stories about "change management." In not one of these stories did the top set bodacious goals or broadcast vision statements, both of which are defining features, by the way, of adolescence. They are not laminating their vision and declaring "infection is not an option." Or claiming "we will 100% eliminate hospital infections by the year 2020." Top management is not needed for inspiration or motivation or role modeling, other than washing their own hands. All that is required is enough support and a little money to allow the process to work.

Most improvement efforts are about profound speaking. And if the message is not working, turn up the volume. PD is only about the listening.

5. *This is a peer-based learning process rather than an expert-based teaching process.* The Highlander Center in Tennessee worked this way in fulfilling a major role in the U.S. civil rights movement. They call this part of the process "popular education." They said their role as educators was to help people discover what they already know. They knew that people on the margin or near the bottom of the social structure did not know their own wisdom. Did not know what they know. PD gets this and takes it to scale. Popular education calls us to find processes where a system discovers what it already knows. This is a relocation of where expertise resides. Again, not a small thing.

6. *Positive Deviance is holistic in its thinking.* It is an elegant integration of common spirit from a wide variety of disciplines or fields of endeavor. It takes the best of experiential education and the study of how adults learn. It learns from sociology and cultural anthropology the power of the group and shifting social norms. It calls on the self-organizing wisdom of complexity theory and the large group methodology of organization development where we know the wisdom that is released when the social system is the focus of attention.

There is a deep influence from philosophy and religion in its choice for humility and its appreciation of how leadership is invisible. The process pays deep respect for the values of medicine, both in its applied science and its passion to heal. The engineer finds a place here in its love for assessment, baseline measures, and evidence of improvement over time. Theatre and improvisation became a way of awakening people across divides in a way that none of them had to defend themselves. Finally these are stories of community organizing: slow, persistent relationship building, awareness building, and celebration.

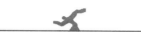

If you want authentic health care reform, the ideas in this book and movement are the portal.

In all these ways the stories here are the face of authentic reform. If you want authentic health care reform, the ideas in this book and movement are the portal. What is also reassuring is that what is uncovered here is occurring in a hundred places. Positive Deviance stands shoulder to shoulder with the amazing work in health care of Paul Uhlig and his commitment to collaborative rounds and its implications. We saw the same values and practices in the Grameen bank in Bangladesh where they extended credit to the poor and created small circles of women creating a new future for themselves.

Dennis Bakke ran a power company on these principles, where, for example, he had local first-line workers manage large financial reserves for local power plants and found they could manage money about as well as their expert-based treasury department. In the field of disabilities there are people like Judith Snow, Al Etmanski, and Joe Erpenbeck who realize that professional services and expertise have serious limits, and we care more deeply when the gifts, desires, humanity, and voices of the disabled are center stage.

At the risk of some repetition, let me offer in more universal language a summary of what PD represents. The following seem to be the strategic elements that are associated with this idea of communal transformation:

- *Choice and Invitation.* The thread in all reform movements is that they are initiated by choice and invitation. They hold deep respect for the presence of local wisdom. They are neurotically wary of experts under any disguise. They allow for local, customized solutions that take advantage of the variability of what it means to be human. Consistency is the problem, not the solution.

- *The End of Ambition.* At the most human level, these reforms are initiated by people at the stage of life where they have given up on ambition. They are often people in midlife, in age or spirit, who reached a point where they are ready to look far outside what they were conditioned and trained in to find meaning for what is to come. Each of these initiators sought, and found, some peace with the suffering and foolishness they were surrounded with for most of their careers.

- *Acts of Dissent.* Healing and reform begins with an act of dissent. Jung said that all consciousness began with an act of disobedience. That act is a betrayal of those that the traditional culture has authorized to speak: the clergy in the church, the physician in medicine, the professor in education, the economist in commerce, the artist in the academy, the consultant in commerce.

- *Gifts and Capacities.* Healing and reform are interested in the gifts and capacities of ordinary people. They are not interested in the gifts of extraordinary people—the world of celebrity, passing fame, and the meta message that this could not happen to you. It is the gifts of those on the margin that change the world. Plus it asks us to finally acknowledge that all this effort in working on deficiencies and needs has not paid dividends. Not for us as individuals nor for all the "poor" countries we give aid to.

- *Community Is It.* Healing and reform is all about a shift or renewal of the collective. Communal transformation. Individuals play a small role in reform. It is when a community, even if just three people, gets organized and determined that health and transformation show up.

- *Humanity Restored.* Finally, reform efforts have to accept the fallibility in each of us. There is great respect for mistakes, which are essential for learning. There is a place for variability, sometimes called diversity. Real reform avoids the instinct for raising the bar, increasing controls, endless automation and the stress on performance. It reclaims and honors our humanity as the ultimate healer. Call it God or spirit, its beliefs rest always on a deep faith in what means to be human.

When you find a method and way of being that holds the promise to pull all of this under one gable, one roof, you pay attention. This, then, is the face of real reform. Reform is about rethinking, in fact inverting, our thinking. What we thought was true turns out to be a story or narrative that was true for a period of time. It just cannot take us any farther. So reform, by its nature, inverts or subverts convention; otherwise it is just an improvement. This work has the potential to jump start, in a supportive and evidence-based way, the real conversation of health care reform that we are seeking. I hope you enjoy the book as much as I did.

Peter Block
July, 2010 Cincinnati, Ohio

Preface

The Daodejing, the work that records treasures of wisdom from ancient China, offered advice for governance, leadership, and change agents. The cryptic and transcendent messages of the text suggested *who leads best meddles least and remains unknown*—and when the tasks of governance are fulfilled people will say, "And with us it happened naturally."

Jerry Sternin, who studied Chinese philosophy at Harvard University and spoke fluent Mandarin, drew inspiration from the poetry and paradox of Daoism and from his own close and empathetic observation of people. Accompanied by his wife, Monique, Jerry's life work involved traveling to dozens of countries on all continents, going to the people—especially the poorest of the poor, the vulnerable, and the marginalized—and living and learning with them. The Sternins started with what people knew, and built on what they had. And, when they left, people had discovered, appropriated, and embodied the wisdom that, to begin with, was their very own.

Positive Deviance (PD) is an approach to social change that enables communities to discover the wisdom they already have, and then to act on it. The premise of PD is that in every community there are certain individuals whose uncommon practices or behaviors enable them to find better solutions to problems than their neighbors who have access to the same resources. These individuals are called "positive" because they were doing things right, and "deviants" because they engaged in behaviors that most others do not. In the PD approach, the role of experts is to help com-

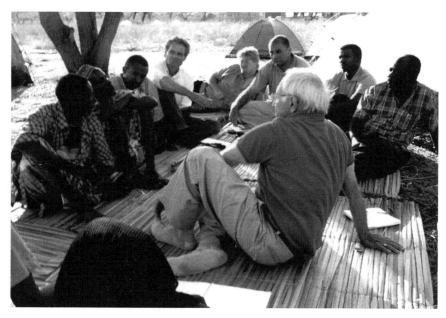

Jerry Sternin (foreground) with Afar elders in Ethiopia

munity members find positive deviants, identify the uncommon but effective things that positive deviants do, and then to make them visible and actionable. PD is led by internal change agents who present the social proof to their peers. Because the PD process amplifies already existing local wisdom, solutions and benefits can be sustained.

The PD Premise:

In every community there are certain individuals whose uncommon practices and behaviors enable them to find better solutions to problems than their neighbors who have access to the same resources.

Jerry and Monique Sternin utilized the PD approach to curb and reduce intractable public health and social problems in several developing countries of Asia, Africa, and Latin America. These include anemia among mothers and children, malnutrition, HIV/AIDS and STDs, female genital cutting, girls trafficking, and the issue of school dropouts.

In the U.S., in more recent years, PD has been used effectively in several health care settings to significantly reduce the incidence of deadly health care-associated infections, especially attributable to an invisible, devious, and deadly bacterium known as MRSA, short for Methicillin-resistant *Staphylococcus aureus*. Health care-associated infections, of which over 60 per cent represent MRSA infections, claim over 100,000 lives each year, more than breast cancer, AIDS, and traffic accidents combined.

This book, *Inviting Everyone: Healing Healthcare through Positive Deviance,* tells the remarkable story of how a people-centered approach to organizational and social change, accompanied by sound scientific and technical expertise, can yield significantly positive quality-of-care outcomes for ordinary citizens, health care institutions, and society in general. In so doing, this work draws upon the collective wisdom and experience of infection control practitioners, medical doctors, public health experts, nurses, social and organizational change practitioners, health care administrators, journalists and writers, and university-based academicians.

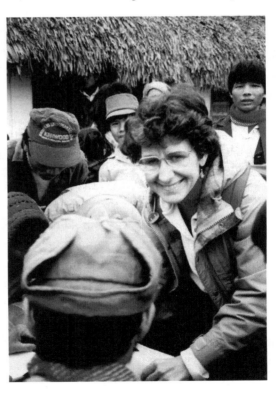

In hospital after hospital, we learned that technical knowledge about infection control was not the main barrier. Doctors and nurses, for instance, knew about appropriate gowning and gloving procedures and necessary hand hygiene protocols. The problem was behavioral: the average hand hygiene compliance rates for health care provider-patient encounters were at 50 per cent or less. The problem was structural: hospitals are disciplinary and specialty

Monique Sternin, working on a childhood malnutrition project in Vietnam silos. The germs, however, know no boundaries. Coffee cups in the hospital cafeteria, housekeeping brooms, doctors' stethoscopes, and nurses' pens all represent vectors of infection. The problem was cultural and relational: for instance, patients find it very difficult to ask their nurse or physician to wash their hands before touching them.

In settings where the PD approach to preventing health care-associated infections yielded significantly positive outcomes, we heard comments such as:

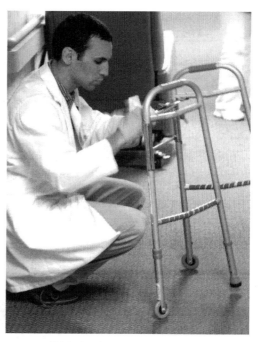

Disinfecting equipment, saving lives at Billings Clinic, Montana

"Lives have been saved in this hospital by changing the way people relate to each other."

"I now feel I have the courage to tell the doctor to gown and glove because we are all collectively responsible for saving patients' lives."

"When infection control is everybody's responsibility, not just the infection control doctor and nurse, then there are thousands of eyes, and hands, and minds working to help, support, and monitor each other."

That is one reason why the title of this book is inclusive: *Inviting Everyone*.

Three days before Jerry Sternin passed away in December 2008, Jon Lloyd, a surgeon and Plexus Institute's Senior Clinical Advisor, visited Jerry in a Boston hospital. Jon had just returned from the recent Institute for Healthcare Improvement National Forum meeting in Nashville, where the hospitals participating in the Positive Deviance approach presented data on statistically significant reductions in MSRA rates, attributable in large measure to the PD processes that were unleashed. "Jerry was unable to speak, but almost busted my hand with a purposeful squeeze when he heard the good news," Jon reported to colleagues in the MRSA initiative. "His eyes projected great pride."

Can the quality of people's lives be improved and can lives be saved by believing in the wisdom of ordinary people? Can the wisdom of ordinary people be unleashed and amplified? Come join this Positive Deviance journey; a journey that made Jerry Sternin visibly proud.

Arvind Singhal, The University of Texas at El Paso, Texas.
Prucia Buscell, Plexus Institute, New Jersey
Curt Lindberg, Plexus Institute, New Jersey

Chapter 1
The People, the Danger and the New Deviants
by Prucia Buscell

There are many gifts that are unique in man; but at the center of them all…lies the ability to draw conclusions from what we see to what we do not see, to move our minds through space and time, and to recognize ourselves in the past on the steps to the present.

— Jacob Bronowski, *The Ascent of Man*

Teri Cartrette had worked in medically related jobs for years and her sister is a nurse. So she knew MRSA infections could be serious. She had just never seen anyone die of one.

She is still haunted by her husband's death in 2006 and the two years of agony that preceded it.

"Unless people have been through this they can't begin to understand the devastation," she said. "I had never seen anything like the way he suffered. None of us had. Our pastor had never seen anything like it either. The infection just wrecked his body. Everything hurt him."

Living a Downward Spiral

Glenn Cartrette had knee surgery in January 2003, recovered quickly and returned to his job as a truck driver. Then he began having pain in his hip that was made worse by long hours behind the wheel. He had hip replacement surgery in October, closely followed by surgical treatment for kidney stones. A stent was inserted into his bladder, and he experienced multiple complications. His health began a downward spiral. Within weeks, his pain was so severe he was unable to continue physical rehabilitation. He began having serious breathing trouble. The couple learned he had a MRSA infection that had traveled to both lungs. Later they were told that Glenn had pulmonary hemosiderosis, a condition in which bleeding and iron build-up in the lungs causes continuing and irreversible damage.

In the following months, Glenn endured repeated emergency hospital admissions and treatments with multiple courses of powerful antibiotics and strong pain medications that left him weak and dazed. For the last seven months of his life, Glenn Cartrette was hospitalized and in relentless pain. Hope for recovery diminished daily. Every breath was a battle. He died on January 26, 2006, at the age of 50. In addition to his widow, he left behind two children and a two month-old grandson. Cartrette says her husband's death certificate lists respiratory failure and MRSA as the cause of death. The financial cost of his ordeal, in hospital bills alone, came to more than $2 million.

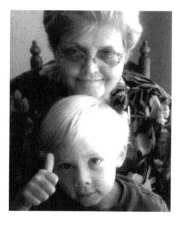

Teri Cartrette's father died 75 days after her husband. He too tested positive for MRSA, though his infection did not cause his death. While her husband and father were ill, her 25-year-old son, who has since recovered, was being treated for cancer with surgery and chemotherapy. All three were in the same hospital. She remembers rushing from one floor to another, always

Teri Cartrette and grandson, Briley, who never got to meet his grandfather donning and removing the gowns, gloves and masks required to go in and out of her husband's isolation room.

Cartrette lives in North Carolina with her sister, who is now retired. She works at a dentist's office during the day, and nights and weekends she is on call for a home health company, talking to patients and dispatching aides. "I am very busy, and I like to be busy because you don't have time to think too much," she said.

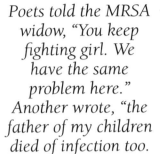

Most of her husband's expenses were covered by insurance. Cartrette had struggled to keep up the $800 a month for his private insurance and some doctor bills. Because he was disabled by his illness, Medicare covered some later expenses. Shortly before his death, she learned he had used up his lifetime Medicare benefits, but would be eligible for Medicaid coverage. Some providers filed claims against his estate, she said, but nothing was left.

Poets told the MRSA widow, "You keep fighting girl. We have the same problem here." Another wrote, "the father of my children died of infection too. Changes need to be made."

"I'd never heard of Medicare just running out," Cartrette said. "You hate to say these aren't my bills when it's someone you love. But no ordinary human being could pay all those bills."

In addition to working as many hours as possible, Cartrette sought solace in poetry. She had always loved reading poetry, and had eclectic tastes that ranged from Rudyard Kipling to Helen Steiner Rice. Trying to heal and make sense of Glenn's inexplicable decline and death, she began putting her own thoughts in poems. She wrote of love, loss, and the disorientation of prolonged sadness. In one poem she touched on how the death of a loved one disrupts a sense of time and tears the film of familiarity from ordinary things. She joined *ThePoetsTree.com*, a website where contributors read and analyze each other's work. In a poem called "We Must Stand," she wrote of her support for state laws requiring public reporting of hospital infections, which she believes would help both hospitals and patients. The poem speaks of faith, and her husband's kindness, and includes the lines:

I will continue to fight for hospitals to share
I want them to rethink some of their care.

This illness you had could have been spared
If those that knew had shown that they cared.

She cited official figures on lives lost to health care-associated infections, then concluded,

You were one in 90,000 to them you see
Yet you were the whole world to me.

More than 50 fellow poets responded. "You keep fighting girl. We have the same problem here," wrote one. Another wrote, "The father of my children died of infection too," wrote another. "Changes need to be made." Several said they had survived MRSA and other infections acquired in hospitals, or lost family members to them. Many thanked her for telling her experience in poetry. Several praised her fortitude and compassion.

Cartrette has written to legislators and contributed her story to web sites that present experiences of patients and families who have coped with hospital infections. Accompanied by her husband's cousin, who is a social worker, she also met with members of the board of the hospital where her husband and father died to urge more attention to infection prevention. The encounter was painful and discouraging. "They didn't understand our purpose. They were just so afraid I was going to sue," she recalled, adding that a lawsuit had never been her intention. "When we tried to talk to them, they kept telling me all the things they thought I had done wrong—that I had denied Glenn medicine when he was in pain. It had gotten to the point Glenn couldn't take more—doctors and nurses agreed about that. Later they (hospital officials) wrote me a letter saying they heard me and were trying to make changes. But basically, they blew us off."[1]

While the very young, the very old and those with compromised immune systems are most susceptible to infection, MRSA is also known to strike adolescent and young adult athletes, soldiers and others in prime physical condition.

Even the Young and Strong Are Vulnerable

Ian Blackwelder had wanted to be a Navy SEAL since the seventh grade. He spent his teen years training—running hills, swimming miles, doing push ups and pull ups. He was an Eagle Scout who worked four summers at Camp Pipsico Boy Scout Camp in Virginia, where he was aquatics director during his last summer. He was in ROTC through high school, which he finished in three years. When he began boot camp in July, 2007 at age 18, he was in excellent physical condition, 6 feet 3 inches tall, and a well-toned 190 pounds. When he caught a cold, no one thought much of it. "People bring their own germs from all over the country, and it winds up combining into what they call 'recruit crud'," Ian Blackwelder remembered. "Everyone gets it, no matter how healthy they are." But the cold didn't get better, and he developed a bad backache.

By his seventh week of boot camp, he was admitted to the North Chicago Veterans Administration hospital intensive care unit. He had pneumonia, sepsis and kidney failure. His mother, Michelle Blackwelder, flew from Virginia. A hospital chaplain met her with the news Ian's survival was in doubt. He was on a ventilator. As next of kin, she had to consent to surgery to drain his lung cavity. A drainage tube inserted under his arm into his chest produced three liters of fluid. The pneumonia that started in

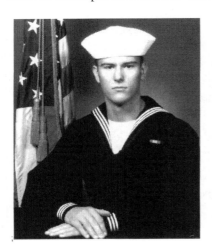

Ian Blackwelder, who entered Naval boot camp at age 18, had trained to be a Navy SEAL since junior high school.

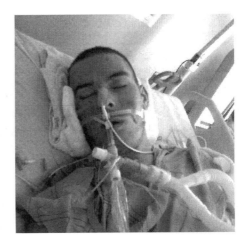

Ian was kept unconscious for 13 days while he was on a ventilator being treated for the MRSA infection that nearly killed him.

one lung had spread to both. His heart was beating too fast, his temperature was too high, and his blood pressure was too low. Doctors told Michelle Blackwelder they weren't sure what organism was causing the pneumonia, information needed for effective treatment. During his 13 days on a ventilator, he was kept unconscious so he wouldn't pull out the tubes.

When Ian caught a cold, no one thought much of it... By his seventh week of boot camp, he was admitted to the intensive care unit.

Michelle Blackwelder called a friend who is a nurse, described everything being done, and named all bags of intravenous fluids and medicines. The friend got the next flight to the hospital. "She told me later that it sounded as though he was dying and she didn't want me to go through that alone," Blackwelder said.

The VA hospital didn't have a thoracic surgeon on staff, so Ian Blackwelder underwent more surgery to remove more fluid building up in his chest at a nearby civilian hospital. After 14 days, he was transferred back to the VA hospital for rehabilitation. Before leaving, his mother noticed that his underarm scar had healed, but the scars from the most recent surgery on his back looked angry and inflamed. A nurse took a culture. In the civilian hospital, he had shared a room with a heart surgery patient. Back at the VA, he was on a rehab floor with many older patients. He made friends with a 75-year-old man. "We were laughing about Bingo and John Wayne movies," his mother recalled. After two or three days, the VA hospital received results of the wound culture. It was positive for MRSA. Ian was put in isolation and started on another round of antibiotics.

Michelle Blackwelder returned to her home and job. A week later, Ian asked her to return. He would need another two weeks of hospital care. When she arrived, on a Friday evening, she was told Ian was being sent back to the Naval recruiting center so their visit would be only a matter of minutes. A naval captain intervened, and said Ian could stay with his mother until 8 PM Sunday. On Saturday morning, Ian showered and asked his mother to put new dressings on the surgical scars on his back. She was shocked by what she saw. "Nothing had healed, and the scars were nasty and oozing pus," Michelle Blackwelder said. "I said we need to take you back to the hospital, but he refused. He said he had already told them how sick he felt, and they hadn't cared."

Ian Blackwelder had started taking sulfa drugs prescribed for the MRSA infections, but no one knew he was allergic to them. By Saturday night, he was covered with hives. He was weak, barely able to stand, and vomiting repeatedly. On Sunday morning, with Ian feverish, Michelle Blackwelder went out and bought a thermometer. She drove Ian back to the VA hospital and by that time his temperature was 104 degrees. His chest cavity was drained again, and this time tests showed MRSA was in the fluid, not just the wounds. A week later, he was released. The illness, infection, the four surgeries and all the medications had taken a heavy physical toll. His weight had dropped to 145 pounds and he was too weak to carry a duffle bag. His 30 days of convalescence turned into 60.

The company that handles military health insurance tells patients what their care cost. In Ian's case, it was $600,000 for one hospital and $400,000 for the other.

His life was changed. His damaged, scarred lungs disqualified him from the Navy SEAL program. He was transferred to an air crew training program in Florida, but did not pass the physical. In February 2009, he was medically discharged from the Navy. His request for disability benefits has been denied, and he has appealed. He thought he might get work scuba diving—which had been his hobby—but his lungs don't work well enough for that, either. Ian Blackwelder turned 21 on April 19, 2010. He is now married and is using his GI education benefits to attend community college. He plans to transfer to a four-year college and is still searching for a new career goal. He is stoic about his physical losses— he says he is now able to run and swim. He has avoided bitterness, he said, "because I have had time to think it about it." But he admits losing some of his youthful optimism and buoyancy: "When I was 18, I was really motivated. I thought people were inherently good."

In retrospect, he feels bad about the heart patient who shared his room while he had the raging MRSA infection, and the older patients with whom he mingled in the VA rehab rooms before his MRSA was identified. He does not know whether they became infected. Michelle Blackwelder remembers using hand gel frequently while Ian was at the civilian hospital. Gowns and gloves were available outside the door, but a nurse told her she didn't have to use them. Both mother and son are shocked by the expense of Ian's inpatient care. The company that handles military health insurance tells patients what their care cost. In Ian's case, it was $600,000 for one hospital and $400,000 for the other. He wonders whether that million dollars and his lungs could have been saved with a few dollars worth of the right antibiotic at the right time.[2]

The Cost of MRSA

Studies on the financial impact of the extra cost of health care-associated (HA) infections vary widely, but the costs are staggering, and always in billions. A study published in the *Archives of Internal Medicine* in 2010 reported that protracted hospital stays and treatment just for patients with HA pneumonias and sepsis, often caused by MRSA and other superbugs, cost $8 billion in 2006.[3] A study for the federal Centers for Disease Control and Prevention (CDC) by economist R. Douglas Scott II, published in 2009, found that the annual direct medical costs of all HA infections to U.S. hospitals for inpatient services, adjusting to 2007 dollars, ranged from $35.7 billion to $45 billion a year. Adjusting for varying effectiveness of differing prevention methods, hospitals could save anywhere from a low of $5.7 billion to $6.8 billion annually for preventing 20 per cent of HA infections, to a high of $25 billion to $31.5 billion if 70 per cent of HA infections were prevented.[4]

The financial waste and personal tragedies of MRSA and other infections leave no doubt that infection control is urgent. Health care professionals know infection prevention protocols. The question is how to implement them consistently. Because this effort involves behavior of huge numbers of people and virtually countless interactions among humans and microbes, the task is much harder than it sounds.

MRSA and many other pathogens are spread by human contact—passed from one person to another by contact with germs on hands, personal items, clothing, and environmental surfaces contaminated with bacteria.

While firm figures are hard to get, several surveys suggest adherence to hand hygiene protocols—hand washing or sanitizing before and after every patient contact—hovers around 50 per cent among clinicians and other health care workers.

Bacterial Ingenuity

The multidisciplinary scholar and author Jared Diamond suggests that to understand disease, we need to put aside our human biases and try to think like a microbe.[5] That's a challenge, because microbes are vastly more numerous, more diverse and eons older than humans. They can live anywhere. Bacteria have been found in boiling hot springs, in freezing seawater and deep beneath the Antarctic ice sheet under subglacial Lake Vostok, one of the most isolated environments on earth. Bacteria have been found deep in volcanic rock, and in the mysterious darkness of the sea floor where many scientists think life began. Some bacteria survive in toxic environments where nothing else lives.[6]

We need to put aside our human biases and try to think like a microbe.

Microbes outnumber and outweigh humans. They comprise 60 per cent of the mass of life on earth and their estimated collective mass is 50 to 60 quadrillion metric tons. The average human may have some 10 trillion cells in the body, but the microbes on and in every living human can number from 50 trillion to 100 trillion.[7]

In fact, humans host teeming communities of microorganisms, some of which are helpful to natural ecological and bodily processes. We wouldn't survive without the bacterial activities that help digestion and the development of the immune system. Some harmless bacteria occupy space that would be invaded by pathogens if not for their presence.

Bacteria do many of the things that humans do. They grow, breathe and communicate. Like military strategists, they know when their collective number has accumulated enough to do real damage. The tiny dose of poison from one bacterial cell wouldn't do much. But bacterial communities have an ability called quorum sensing that allows them to signal for the release of disease-causing toxins when their numbers reach critical mass. Princeton biologist Bonnie Bassler has even found signaling mechanisms that enable bacteria to communicate with species other than their own, allowing them to swap genetic information helpful to adapting and mutating. She calls it "bacterial Esperanto."[8]

Bacteria evolve. Just like human populations, successful bacteria reproduce efficiently and find good places to live. Diamond explains success for a disease-causing microbe means finding a suitable host victim and infecting as many new victims as possible. It isn't really in the microbe's interest to kill us. A patient's death, in the microbial view, is just collateral damage. In fact, if the patient lives to get sick and spread germs again, that's better for the microbe. Diamond says "we and our pathogens are now in an escalating evolutionary contest with the death of one contestant the price of defeat and with natural selection playing the role of umpire."[9]

In Roman times when world trade routes linked populations and con-

Ignaz Semmelweis and Invisible Cadaveric Particles

In 1847, a 29-year-old Hungarian doctor, Ignaz Phillip Semmelweis, working as a midwifery physician in Vienna's General Hospital, became intrigued by a puzzling statistic: the hospital ward in which physicians delivered babies had three times the maternal mortality rate of the ward where the midwives were in charge.[1] The cause of these maternal deaths was attributed to puerperal fever, also called childbed fever, a disease common in mid-nineteenth century European hospitals. As many as 35 per cent of its victims died.

Semmelweis also noticed that the obstetric physicians and their trainees spent their morning dissecting cadavers of patients who had died of puerperal fever. Then they conducted routine examinations of their living patients, probing the uterus, cervix, and womb with bare unwashed hands. If a new baby needed to be delivered, it was often done with the same unclean hands. While unthinkable today, in the mid-nineteenth century this was fairly common practice, because many medical authorities still thought disease was caused by "bad air" and imbalanced bodily "humors" of individuals. While Antony van Leeuwenhoek, inventor of the microscope, reported in the late 1600s that he saw "little living animalcules" in lake water and bodily fluids, it would be years before scientists related this microscopic life to disease.[2] Semmelweis hypothesized that "cadaveric particles" introduced into the women during examinations and delivery caused puerperal fever, and that infectious agents were spread through the hands of the physicians.

When Semmelweis implemented rigorous hand-washing and scrubbing procedure in the doctors' ward, most notably

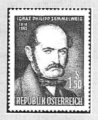

An Austrian stamp honoring Semmelweis

tagious illnesses of Europe, Asia and North Africa, Diamond points out that pathogens flourished and traveled along with commerce. Many scholars say today's ease of global human travel intensifies the universal threat of well-traveled infectious agents. An international research team recently tracked a virulent strain of MRSA that traveled from Europe to South America and Asia. During its journey, the strain, which resists almost every known antibiotic, continued to evolve and was reintroduced into Europe.[10] Jiah-Shin The and Harvey Rubin, two University of Pennsylvania scholars with expertise in infectious disease and bio-security, say experts fear epi-

with chloride of lime solutions, a powerful antiseptic, the incidence of puerperal fever dropped precipitously from 17 per cent of all patients to one per cent.

While many hailed Semmelweis as the "savior of mothers", the medical establishment of the time shunned Semmelweis and others who believed in disease-causing germs and derided his ideas of infection control. Puerperal fever, and the accompanying deaths, was accepted as the price of delivering babies. Oliver Wendell Holmes, the American physician and poet, had argued in 1843 that puerperal fever was contagious, and spread by physicians, though he did not focus on hand hygiene.[3] Holmes too was ridiculed for his contagion theory, but he fared better than Semmelweis, who was dismissed from the hospital in Vienna. Semmelweis moved to Budapest, where he continued his campaign for hand hygiene. He may have suffered a nervous breakdown. His contemporaries and family believed he was losing his mind, and he was committed to a mental institution, where he died of injuries and, ironically, in-

fection. Semmelweis' strict hand-hygiene protocols would gain credibility two decades later when the French chemist and microbiologist Louis Pasteur confirmed the germ theory of disease.

Notes

1. David Cohn, "Semmelweis," University of Louisville. http://pyramid.spd.louisville.edu/~eri/fos/semmelweis.htmlSemmelweis, (accessed 6-29-10); and Irvine Loudon, "Semmelweis and his Thesis," *Journal of the Royal Society of Medicine*, vol. 98 no. 2. http://www.ncbi.nlm.nih.gov/pmc/articles/PMC1299347/ (accessed 6-16-10).

2. Ben Waggoner, "Antony van Leeuwenhoek," University of California Museum of Paleontology. http://www.ucmp.berkeley.edu/history/leeuwenhoek.html; (accessed 5-10-10).

3. Wikipedia, "Oliver Wendell Holmes, Sr." http://en.wikipedia.org/wiki/Oliver_Wendell_Holmes,_Sr. (accessed 5-5-10).

demics of contagious illnesses caused by bacteria that resist every known antibiotic. They assert many medical authorities think antibiotic resistance is the most serious problem facing the medical community today.[11]

Emerging Pestilence

MRSA is a classic case of increasing and evolving resistance. The CDC estimates that in 2005 nearly 100,000 people developed serious MSRA infections, and about 18,650 of them died during a hospital stay related to the infection.[12] MRSA is one of the most common health care infections, and most of those documented by the CDC were identified as health care-associated (HA). But community-associated (CA) MRSA infections that often cause skin lesions and abscesses among otherwise healthy people who have not been recently treated in health care facilities, are increasingly turning up in hospitals. That worries doctors, because while both HA and CA MRSA can cause serious illness and death, there is some evidence that community strains, which differ genetically from HA MRSA and seem to have arisen separately, may be more virulent.[13]

Bacteria began developing resistance to antibiotics just a few years after penicillin, first used in 1941, began saving lives. Methicillin was introduced in 1961, and resistance began shortly thereafter, giving a hint of bacterial resilience and ingenuity. Because Methicillin was based on penicillin, researchers thought *staph* bacteria would resist it in the same way. Instead, the bacteria found a new way. Penicillin weakened the structure of the *staph* cell walls, and the resistant bacteria learned to disable that mechanism. *Staph* bacteria resistant to Methicillin evolved in ways that protected its cell walls and left Methicillin unable to damage them.[14]

Differing strains of MRSA are now resistant to many antibiotics, and have many mechanisms for evading or defeating medicines designed to kill them. Antibiotic resistance burgeoned as more people used more antibiotics, and the development of new antibiotics has not kept pace. Patients demanded a pill for more ailments, and doctors prescribed more antibiotics for more ills, including viruses, against which they have no effect. Patients often didn't finish their antibiotic course, leaving their own disease-causing bacteria hardier. The extensive use of antibiotics in agriculture and animal feed augmented the trend.

Some *staph aureus* strains are even developing resistant to Vancomycin, a drug commonly known as a last resort for patients with MSRA infections that are not susceptible to any other antibiotic. That keeps doctors awake at night.

Some alarming facts about MRSA and other health care-associated infections include the following:

- Among the 2.1 million people in the U.S. who acquired infections while hospitalized in 2000, nearly 100,000 died.[15]

Bonnie Bassler has found signaling mechanisms that enable bacteria to communicate with other species, allowing them to swap genetic information helpful to adapting. She calls it "bacterial Esperanto."

- Health care-associated infections are one of the most serious patient safety concerns and merit urgent attention, according to the 2009 *National Health Care Quality Report* from the U.S. Agency for Healthcare Research and Quality. The report says progress on health care-associated infections is lagging, with post operative sepsis, or blood infections, worsening at the fastest rate.[16]

- Hospitals are prone to become reservoirs for MRSA and other resistant pathogens because so many strains of bacteria coexist with so many antibiotics, and so many health care professionals, staff members, patients and visitors move about in such close quarters. The ecology of microorganisms—the bacteria, viruses, fungi and protozoa—in a health care environment is a daunting challenge to infection control.

- In 2002 an estimated 100 million people carried *staph aureus* harmlessly in their noses and three million of them carried the drug resistant variety. A CDC survey finished in 2004 showed a decline in carriers—from 32.4 per cent of the population to 28.6 per cent—but an increase in the drug resistant variety that was carried. The portion of the population carrying MRSA in their noses rose from 0.8 per cent to 1.5 per cent. That change sounds slight, but 1.5 per cent of the population in 2004 was 4.38 million. Some people carry MRSA in body crevices other than their noses, so these numbers may be understated.[17]

- MRSA is a sturdy organism that can also live on hard environmental surfaces, and on soft surfaces, for days and months, depending on temperature, humidity and other conditions.

Serendipity and Emergence: A Messy Lab, a Moldy Cantaloupe and a Scientific Breakthrough

Alexander Fleming, a bacteriologist at St. Mary's Hospital in London, wasn't known for keeping a tidy lab, and it turns out that was lucky for future generations. In 1928, returning from a vacation, he saw mold growing on the plates where he had been culturing *Staphylococcus aureus*. Then he noticed something odd: the mold was surrounded by a visual halo—a clear space with no bacteria. Something about the mold was stopping bacterial growth. He isolated an extract from the mold and called it Penicillium.

His findings, published in a 1929 paper, were part of the extraordinary series of events that led to penicillin, the lifesaving drug that revolutionized medical care. George Wong, an associate professor of botany at the University of Hawaii, tells the remarkable story of how ancient notions and modern research coalesced in the emergence of a twentieth century medical miracle. Fleming served in the British Army Medical Corps in World War I, and he had seen soldiers die of infections after successful surgeries. He suspected antiseptics used during and after surgery might harm immune cells more than disease cells, so he began looking for new ways to kill bacteria. The ancients had used fermented materials and mold-containing earth to heal infections, with some success, so they may have unknowingly used crude preparations similar to antibiotics.[1]

In 1895 a French physician, Ernest Duchesne, discovered that a Penicillium mold stopped growth of the intestinal *E. coli* bacteria.[2] In 1922, Fleming had discovered lysosyme, an enzyme in egg whites, tears, and mucus. Experimenting with mucus from his own nose, he found the enzyme could kill weak bacteria. So he knew that bacteria-free halo around the Penicillium mold was highly significant. But no one knew how to produce Penicillium in quantity, and Fleming turned to other interests.[3]

Years later, one of Fleming's former students, Cecil Paine, successfully treated patients with a small amount of Penicillium mold extract. He may have discussed his experience with Howard Florey, a pathology professor who had read Fleming's paper. Florey had a well-equipped lab and a team of scientists at Oxford, where development of penicillin was in progress. But scaling up was an obstacle. Wong notes that in 1940 it took two professors, five graduate students, and ten assistants working every day for months to get enough penicillin to treat six patients. By

- Some 126,000 people are hospitalized with MSRA infections annually, and people with MRSA infections are four times more likely to die than patients with *staph aureus* infections that are susceptible to antibiotics.

1941, Florey and a colleague Norman Heatley, supported by the Rockefeller Foundation, went to the U. S. Department of Agriculture Northern Laboratory in Peoria, Illinois, to get help.[4]

Working with Andrew J. Moyer, the lab's expert on the nutrition of molds, the scientists were able to increase the yield ten-fold by culturing Penicillium in corn liquor. But they still couldn't produce a practical amount. Then, the USDA reports, the agricultural scientists made a breakthrough. They found a superior strain of Penicillium on a moldy cantaloupe in a Peoria garbage can. When drug companies got the new strain, production soared. Penicillin became available to treat wounded soldiers who survived D-Day, the June 6, 1944 Allied invasion of Normandy, and it has saved countless lives in the decades that followed. Medical researchers began an intensive search for more antimicrobial agents, which would eventually be found not only among molds but even more among bacterial strains themselves.[5]

Fleming was knighted, along with Florey, in 1944, and in 1945 Fleming, Florey, and Ernst Boris Chain, a scientist who worked at Oxford with Florey after fleeing Nazi Germany, received the Nobel Prize for medicine. Ironically, Fleming was beginning to realize a potential danger:

that bacterium would eventually recombine genetically to become resistant to penicillin and other antibiotics.[6]

In 1987, Andrew Moyer, PhD, was posthumously inducted to the National Inventors Hall of Fame in Virginia, joining the ranks of Thomas Edison and the Wright Brothers. He was the first government scientist to be so honored.

Notes
1. George Wong, "The Story of Penicillin, Wonder Drug," University of Hawaii at Manoa, Botany. http://www.botany.hawaii.edu/faculty/wong/BOT135/Lect21b.htm (accessed 11/15/09).

2. Jessica Snyder Sachs, *Good Germs, Bad Germs, Health and Survival in a Bacterial World*, (New York: Hill and Wang 2010), 31.

3. Wong, "The Story of Penicillin." USDA, Agricultural Research Service, "The Rescue of Penicillin." http://www.ars.usda.gov/is/timeline/penicillin.htm, 6/06/08, (accessed 11-09-09).

4. Ibid.

5. David Ho, "The Time 100, Alexander Fleming." http://205.188.238.181/time/time100/scientist/profile/fleming.html (accessed 3-5-10).

6. Ibid.

- Surgical patients, especially those who have joint replacements and heart value replacements, are among the most vulnerable to health care-associated infections.

- Community-associated MRSA is genetically different from health care-associated MRSA, and seems to have arisen separately. While it is generally associated with skin and soft tissue afflictions, it can be deadly. It is known to strike otherwise healthy young people who have not been in a health care facility.

Hospitals are prone to become reservoirs for MRSA and other resistant pathogens because so many strains of bacteria coexist with so many antibiotics, and so many health care professionals, staff members, patients and visitors move about in such close quarters.

- MRSA and other pathogens have a host of tools to cause human disease. They can secrete numerous toxins that damage human cells and disable white blood cells, and produce enzymes that help them evade immune cells.

When bacteria get inside the body, the result is a complex interplay between invader and host. "The body basically goes to war, and it has various ways to do that," explains John Jernigan, MD, MS, deputy chief of the Prevention and Response Branch, in the CDC's Division of Healthcare Quality Promotion. "As part of the immune response, the body can track cells to the area of infection, and these cells produce substances designed to fight the bacteria. If these substances are not produced in the correct amounts or are not properly balanced with one another, they can have deleterious effects on human tissue. For reasons we don't understand, the immune response can occasionally be over-exuberant and cause as much harm to the host as the invader does."[18]

Researchers aren't sure why MRSA strikes different people in different ways—why some infections impact bones and joints and others impact organs. The result of any bacterial invasion depends on the bacteria and its host. "Many bacteria have the machinery to produce various proteins and other chemical factors that help them survive and cause damage within the body," Jernigan said. "Bacteria can also change once they are inside the body. Outside the body they can have a certain set of machinery at work, and gaining access to the inside of the body results in activation of other machinery that can contribute to a harmful effect. They have toolsets that can change depending on the environments in which they find themselves."

Just as ancient trade routes helped traveling microbes spread new disease, a tube placed directly into the blood stream or urinary tract, or any normally sterile bodily space, creates a highway for hostile bacteria to enter the innermost recesses. Jernigan said any kind of foreign object in the body—artificial joints, metal screws, prosthetic devices—make it easier for bacteria to survive and evade the immune system and action of antibiotics. He said many bacteria have the ability to form self-protective biofilms and change their metabolism in ways that make it harder for antibiotics to work. Further, he said, it takes fewer bacteria to cause infection in the presence of a foreign object, and *staph aureus* is one invader that is particularly adept at causing infection around prosthetic devices. "When that happens, you're behind the eight ball," he said. "The chance of a cure with antibiotic therapy alone drops, and you have to remove the device to successfully treat the infection. When you are talking about a prosthetic joint or a heart valve, that's a big deal."

Increasing drug resistance in many important health care pathogens is a vicious cycle, Jernigan said. Infections from resistant organisms require broader spectrum antibiotics, which increases the antimicrobial pressure being exerted on the bacterial ecology as a whole. Bacteria learn to resist more antibiotics. "We have some very multi-resistant bacteria that have very few, if any, options for treatment, and we are pulling some very old very toxic drugs off the shelf," he said. Narrow spectrum antibiotics can treat antibiotic susceptible organisms, and that helps to reduce the trend toward resistance. He said there isn't much data showing reversals in development of resistance.

"We've seen promising data in terms of preventing some infections," he said. "The rate of blood stream associated catheter infections is down. That's good." However, he notes the prevention of those infections requires interventions that avert infections from the germs people already carry. They are not designed to prevent transmission of germs from one person to another.

The Positive Deviance Effect

Positive Deviance was first used to address intractable health and social problems in the developing world. PD pioneers Jerry and Monique Sternin helped bring the concept to U.S. hospitals in workshops and small pilot projects 2004 and 2005. Discussions among hospital executives and quality improvement staff connected with Plexus Institute, and CDC experts and leaders from Plexus Institute and the Positive Deviance Initiative at Tufts University, led to a collective realization that something new was needed in infection prevention. While prevention protocols had been known for more than a century, adherence was an unrelenting challenge. Experience led these colleagues to believe that the engagement of an entire hospital community is needed to halt the spread of infection, and that social and behavioral change are essential if the known technical solutions are to be consistently practiced.

In 2006 The Robert Wood Johnson Foundation awarded a $294,000 grant for an effort led by Plexus Institute and the Positive Deviance Initiative to use a PD approach to fight MRSA. The idea is that PD, which does not rely on new drugs or technology, encourages the kinds of cultural changes that energize people for the task of making infection prevention practices universal and habitual. Six hospitals in the U.S. and two in South America joined the initial Plexus PD MRSA Prevention Partnership.

Beta Site hospitals in the partnership were:

- Albert Einstein Medical Center, Philadelphia, PA

- Billings Clinic, Billings, MT

- Franklin Square Hospital Center, Baltimore, MD

- The Johns Hopkins Hospital, Baltimore, MD

- University of Louisville Hospital, Louisville, KY

- Veterans Administration Pittsburgh Healthcare System, Pittsburgh, PA

- Hospital El Tunal, Bogota, Colombia

- Hospital Pablo Tobon Uribe, Medellin, Colombia

Partnership hospitals agreed to:

- Test all patients in pilot units to find whether they were infected or colonized with MRSA. "Colonization" means a person carries the bacteria but has no symptoms.

- Place all patients carrying or infected with MRSA in isolation and contact precautions—no one enters their rooms without gowns and gloves.

- Promote consistent hand hygiene.

- Report all MRSA infections to the CDC through the National Health-care Safety Network.

- Use Positive Deviance to engage everyone in MRSA prevention.

The Positive Deviance interventions focused on preventing transmission, which Jernigan says is important for two reasons. First of all, it prevents infection. But in addition, the epidemiology of susceptible strains of MRSA may be different from the epidemiology of resistant strains. The presence of resistant strains may be more likely to be the result of transmission. Patients infected with resistant strains don't do as well. They are sick longer and are harder to treat. Interestingly, Jernigan added, the resistant strains of *staph auerus* actually may be less fit for survival, so if they are prevented from spreading, their overall prevalence is reduced relative to more sensitive strains.

"If you shut down transmission," he said, "the antibiogram gets better."

That happened early in the intervention in three of the hospitals in the PD MRSA Prevention Partnership. Declines in *staph aureus* infections were accompanied by declines in the percentage of other infections caused by the drug-resistant microbes. The antibiogram is the result of laboratory tests that determine the susceptibility of a certain pathogen to antibiotics.

"If the results of these three hospitals can be sustained and replicated," Jernigan said, "the implications are huge."

In addition to MRSA, prevalent resistant pathogens include *Klebsiela pneumoniae*, which has epidemiologists in the U.S. and Colombia worried. *Acinetobactor* infections that afflicted soldiers returning from Iraq are increasingly prevalent in U.S. hospitals, and *Clostridium difficile*, a multi drug resistant pathogen that can cause deadly diarrhea, is a growing concern. Infections caused by C-diff have increased every year since 2007, and in some hospitals are more prevalent than MRSA.[19]

"I am very anxious to see if some of the principles we have applied against MRSA can be applied against other resistant organisms for which transmission plays an important role—including the ones that are very difficult to treat except with the older very toxic agents," Jernigan said.

Some infection control authorities think it is unwise for prevention initiatives to focus on one pathogen. They fear the narrow focus will mean other pathogens will get less vigilance, and they want to concentrate on the infections caused by germs people already carry. Jernigan is convinced good programs can prevent infections from germs individuals already carry and prevent transmissions too. "It's not either or," he said. "It's hard. But we can do both."

"If the results of these three hospitals can be sustained and replicated," Jernigan said, *"the implications are huge."*

He adds that infection fighting has to be a regional and community effort. "If we want to control infections by preventing transmission," he said, "then all health care facilities that share patients are in this together. And we won't be really effective until all are making these efforts. We are all dependent on one another."

If fewer people carrying or infected with MRSA come to hospitals, the MRSA prevalence in hospitals will decline. Figures show there has been some decline in MRSA prevalence among people admitted to Veterans Administration hospitals and hospitals in the PD MRSA Partnership.

Jernigan said in 14 VA hospitals examined by the CDC, MRSA colonization ranged from 9 to 27 per cent among people admitted to long-term care, and 9 to 16 per cent among people admitted to intensive care units and medical wards, and those rates are declining. The PD Partnership hospitals began with MRSA prevalence rates ranging from 12 to 20 per cent among ICU admissions, and that has declined to prevalence rates that range from 6 to 18 per cent. In effect, he emphasizes, health care organizations that prevent transmissions and infections are helping all patients, not just their own.

Successful infection fighting means mobilizing every person in a health care environment, and the use of PD processes has been found to foster engagement in communities and organizations. People who help find solutions to workplace problem are often more committed to carrying them out, and organizational culture changes. As a respiratory therapist at Albert Einstein Medical Center observed, one little slip-up can undermine the most careful infection prevention plans, so it's important for people to help each other stay alert to avoiding all contamination possibilities. New relationships develop as people collaborate across different disciplines within organizations, and those internal networks often expand beyond the walls of any one health care organization. In the case of the PD MRSA Prevention Partnership, relationships forged in an initial assault on MRSA infections have continued and expanded, with new participants collaborating for new goals. The overarching goal, however, remains. Those who have seen the ravages of infection want to end the bodily wreckage that led to Glenn Cartrette's death, and damaged Ian Blackwelder's lungs and ended his boyhood dream of being a Navy SEAL.

The following chapters discuss both practical and intangible aspects of the PD process. They cover the Sternin's work in Vietnam and other developing countries. Stories from the PD MRSA Prevention Partnership hospitals illustrate the flexibility and strength of PD as it has been adapted to new environments. The health care workers whose courage and commitment to patient care led them to try a new approach to infection prevention tell of their early frustration, surprising experiences, and their success against a deadly pathogen. Facilitators experienced with PD in health care reflect on the changes they observed in hospitals and in themselves.

Endnotes

1. Interviews with Teri Cartrette, 6-29-09, 11-17-09, 3-17-10.

2. Interviews with Michelle Blackwelder and Ian Blackwelder, 4-29-10.

3. *Medical News Today*, "Hospital Acquired Infections, MRSA killed 48,000 Americans in One Year," 3-23-10, report from February 22 *Archives of Internal Medicine*. http://www.medicalnewstoday.com/articles/180065.php (accessed 4-17-10).

4. Douglas R. Scott, "The Direct Medical Costs of Healthcare-Associated Infections in US Hospitals and the Benefit of Prevention," (Washington: DC, March 2009).

5. Jarred Diamond, *Guns, Germs and Steel: The Fates of Human Societies*. (New York/London: W.W. Norton & Co., 1999), 198-201.

6. Thomas Brock, University of Wisconsin, "Brave New Biosphere," University of Wisconsin-Madison, 1999, http://whyfiles.org/022critters/hot_bact.html (accessed 3-30-10); Tom D'Elia, et al., "Isolation of Lake Vostok Accretion Ice," *Applied and Environmental Microbiology*, vol. 74, no. 15, 4962-4965, http://www.ncbi.nlm.nih.gov/pmc/articles/PMC2519340/pdf/2501-07.pdf (accessed 6-7-10); Laura Urban, "Tough Microbes to Treat Toxins?" *The Scientist, Magazine of Life Sciences,* April 20, 2010, http://www.the-scientist.com/blog/display/57342 (accessed 6-2-10).

7. Brad Spellberg, *Rising Plague: The Global Threat from Deadly Bacteria and Our Dwindling Arsenal to Fight Them,* (Amherst, NY: Prometheus Books, 2009), 98.

8. Bonnie Bassler, "HHMI Scientist Bio: Bonnie L. Bassler, PhD," Howard Hughes Medical Institute, Biomedical Research & Science Education. http://www.hhmi.org/research/investigators/bassler_bio.html (accessed 6-7-10).

9. Diamond, *Guns, Germs and Steel,* 198-201.

10. Rockefeller University, The Rockefeller University Newswire, "Researchers track evolution and spread of drug-resistant bacteria across hospitals and continents." http://newswire.rockefeller.edu/?page=engine&id=1024, Jan 22, 2010, (accessed 4-6-10).

11. Walter Kunreuther and Michael Useem, *Learning From Catastrophes: Strategies for Reaction and Response,* (Upper Saddle River, NJ: Wharton School Publishing, 2010), 219.

12. CDC, "Invasive MRSA," Centers for Disease Control and Prevention. http://www.cdc.gov/ncidod/dhqp/ar_mrsa_Invasive_FS.html (accessed 12-24-09)

13. CDC, Healthcare-Associated *Staphylococus aureus*, Overview of Healthcare Associated MRSA," Centers for Disease Control and Prevention. http://www.cdc.gov/ncidod/dhqp/ar_mrsa.html (accessed 4-17-10).

14. Maryn McKenna, *Superbug: The Fatal Menace of MRSA,* (New York: Simon and Schuster, 2010), 51-52.

15. L.R. Peterson, et al., "New Technology for Detecting Multi-resistant Pathogens in the Clinical Microbiology Laboratory," *Emerging Infections Disease*, vol. 7, no. 2, 306-311.

16. Agency for Healthcare Research Quality (AHRQ), "2009 National Healthcare Quality." http://www.ahrq.gov/qual/nhqr09/Key.htm (accessed 6-8-10).

17. Interviews with Dr. John Jernigan, 8-13-09, 11-4-09; and McKenna, *Superbug,* 83.

18. Interviews with Dr. Jernigan in 2008 and 2009.

19. Duke Medical News and Communications, "New Superbug Surpasses MRSA Infection Rates in Community Hospitals," http://www.dukehealth.org/health_library/news/new_superbug_surpasses_mrsa_infection_rates_in_community_hospitals (accessed 4-17-10).

Chapter 2
Positive Deviance Makes Inroads into Health Care
by Arvind Singhal, Karen Greiner, and Lucia Dura

What is here when the snow covers a thousand mountains?
A single peak not white.

—Ranetsu

The Positive Deviance (PD) approach to social and organizational change is rooted in the water-logged rice fields of northern Vietnam in the 1990s. It spread to other countries of Asia, Africa, and Latin America in the following years, and found its way into the concrete silos of hospitals in the Americas, beginning in 2004. Here is the story of how Jerry and Monique Sternin pioneered PD processes to combat child malnutrition in Vietnam, and then to control and prevent health care-associated infections in the United States and Colombia.

Hanoi, Vietnam; December, 1990

"Sternin, you have six months to show results," said Mr. Nuu, a high-ranking official in the Vietnamese Ministry of Foreign Affairs.

"What? Six months? Six months to demonstrate impact?" Jerry Sternin could not believe his ears.

"Yes, Sternin, six months to show impact, or else I will not be able to extend your visa."

In December, 1990, Jerry Sternin, accompanied by his wife Monique and ten-year old son Sam, arrived in Hanoi to open an office for Save the Children, a U.S.-based non-governmental organization (NGO). His mission: To implement a large-scale program to combat childhood malnutrition in a country where two-thirds of all children under the age of five were malnourished.

The Vietnamese government had learned from experience that results achieved by traditional supplemental feeding programs were not sustainable. When the programs ended, the gains usually tapered off. The Sternins had to come up with an approach that enabled the community, without much outside help, to take control of children's nutritional status.

And quickly! Mr. Nuu had given the Sternins six months!

Crisis or Opportunity

> *There's nothing so practical as a good theory.*[1]
> – Kurt Lewin, pioneer of social psychology

Necessity is the mother of invention. If old methods of combating malnutrition would not yield quick and sustainable results, the Sternins wondered if the construct of Positive Deviance, developed a few years earlier by Tufts University nutrition professor Marian Zeitlin, might hold promise.[2]

The concept of Positive Deviance had entered nutritional literature in the 1960s. Marian Zeitlin explored the idea in some depth in the 1980s as she tried to understand why some children in poor households, without access to any special resources, were better nourished than others. What did they know, and what were they doing that others were not? Perhaps combating malnutrition called for an assets-based approach: that is, iden-

tifying what's going right in a community and finding ways to am
as opposed to the more traditional deficit-based approach of focu
what's going wrong in a community and fixing it.

Positive deviance is an approach to social change that enables communities to discover the wisdom they already have and then to act on it.

The Weight of 2,000 Children and a Mystery Unveiled

Positive Deviance sounded good in theory. But no one to date had used it to actually
design a field-based nutrition intervention.
Might it work in a community setting? How?
The Sternins had no roadmaps or blueprints
to consult. Where to begin?

Positive deviance is an approach to social change that enables communities to discover the wisdom they already have and then to act on it.

Starting close to Hanoi, their home base,
made sense. Childhood malnutrition rates
were high in the Quong Xuong District in
Thanh Hoa Province, south of Hanoi. After a bumpy four-hour ride on
Highway 1 in a black Russian car powered by a noisy tractor engine, the
Sternins arrived on locale. The Ho Chi Minh trail, as Americans call it, was
a supply route for the guerilla fighters during the Vietnam War. It snakes through Quong Xuong, where suspicion of Americans was palpably high. The trail is an extraordinary network of roads, bicycle paths, waterways, and hidden tunnels that passes between North and South Vietnam and through Laos and Cam-

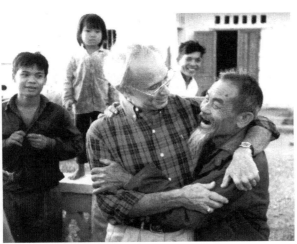

Building Trust: Jerry Sternin with a village elder in Quong Xuong District, Vietnam

bodia. Its history and

legend are seared into American and Vietnamese consciousness. The Sternins first task was to build trust with community members. The rest would follow.

After several days of consultation with local officials, four village communities were selected for a nutrition baseline survey. Armed with six weighing scales and bicycles, health volunteers weighed some 2,000 children under the age of three in four villages, in a record three and a half days. A growth card for each child with a plot of the child's age and weight was created. Some 64 per cent of the weighed children were found to be malnourished.

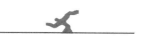

If the community self-discovered the solution, they were more likely to implement it.

No sooner was the data tallied, than with bated breath, the Sternins asked: "Are there any well-nourished children who come from very, very poor families?"

The response: "Yes, yes, there are some children from very, very poor families who are healthy!"

Yes, yes, there are some children from very, very poor families who are healthy!

Workers have labored in rice fields for thousands of years. In Vietnamese literature, the fields are described as wide enough for the wing span of a flock of storks. They are very much a part of Vietnamese life. They are beautiful, and they need constant care, collaboration and ingenuity—the very things needed to both maintain and change culture.

These poor families in Thanh Hoa who had managed to avoid malnutrition without access to any special resources would represent the positive deviants: "positive" because their children were well nourished, and "deviant" because they were doing some things differently.

What were these PD families doing that others were not? To answer this question, community members visited six of the poorest families with well-nourished children in each of the four villages. The Sternins believed that if the community members self-discovered the solution, they were more likely to implement it.

Their discovery process yielded the following key PD practices among poor households with well-nourished children:

- Family members collected tiny shrimps and crabs from paddy fields and added them to their children's meals. These foods are rich in protein and minerals.

- Family members added greens of sweet potato plants to their children's meals. These greens are rich in beta carotene and other essential micronutrients such as iron and calcium.

Interestingly, these foods were accessible to everyone, but most community members believed they were inappropriate for young children. Further:

A thousand hearings isn't worth one seeing, and a thousand seeings isn't worth one doing.

- PD mothers were feeding their children three to four times a day, rather than the customary twice a day.

- PD mothers were actively feeding their children, rather than placing food in front of them, making sure there was no food wasted.

- PD mothers washed the hands of the children before and after they ate.

Doing, Not Telling

With the secrets discovered, the natural urge was to go out and tell the people what to do. Various ideas for "telling" were brainstormed: household visits, attractive posters, and educational sessions, among others. However, from past experience in other countries, the Sternins knew that old habits die hard and new ones, even when they hold obvious advantages, are hard to cultivate. Their experience suggested that such "best practice" solutions almost always engendered resistance from the people. The Sternins coined a phrase for it—the "natural human immune response."

As the discussion wound down, a skeptical village elder observed, "A thousand hearings isn't worth one seeing, and a thousand seeings isn't worth one doing."

On the car ride back to Hanoi, the Sternins talked about the sagacity of the elder's remark. Could they help design a nutrition program that emphasized doing more than seeing or hearing?

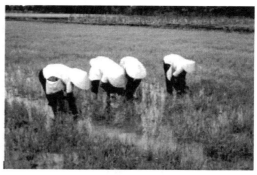

Shrimps and crabs for the taking in Vietnamese rice paddies

A two-week nutrition program was designed with community members in each of the four intervention villages. Mothers whose children were malnourished were asked to forage for shrimps, crabs, and sweet potato greens. Armed with small nets and containers, mothers waded into the paddy fields. The focus was on action, picking up the shrimps and crabs, and shoots from sweet potato fields.

In the company of positive deviants, mothers of malnourished children learned how to cook new recipes using the foraged ingredients. Again, the emphasis was on doing.

Before these mothers fed their children, they weighed them, and plotted the data points on their growth chart. The children's hands were washed, and the mothers actively fed the children. No food was wasted. Some mothers noted their children seemed to eat more in the company of other children. When returning home, mothers were encouraged to give their children three or four small meals a day instead of the traditional two meals.

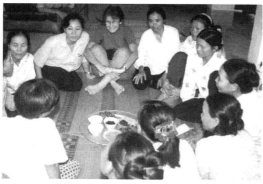

A cooking session in progress in an intervention village

Such feeding and monitoring continued for two weeks. Mothers could visibly see their children becoming healthier. The scales were tipping. And the rest is history.

Positive Deviance as a change process is completely informed by, and bathed in, data. Data are collected at every step of the

way and openly posted for the community members to monitor pro⌐
Data identify where problems and the solutions lie.

After the pilot project, which lasted two years, malnutrition had decreased by an amazing 85 per cent in the PD communities. Over the next
several years, the PD intervention became a nationwide program in Vietnam, helping over 2.2 million people, includ-
ing over 500,000 children improve their
nutritional status. Later studies by Emory
University researchers showed successive
generations of impoverished Vietnamese children in the program villages were well nourished.[3]

Born out of necessity, this pioneering PD
experience in Vietnam, with all its struggles
and lessons, yielded several key insights.
Conventional learning theories assume that
knowledge will change attitudes, which will
in turn change practice. With PD, that idea is
reversed. PD practitioners have found action
is the first step in changing attitudes.

In Jerry Sternin's words, "it is easier to act
your way into a new way of thinking than to
think your way into a new way of acting."

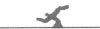

*Positive Deviance
as a change process
is completely informed
by, and bathed in,
data. Data are
collected at every step
of the way and openly
posted for the
community members
to monitor progress.
Data identify where
problems and the
solutions lie.*

Positive Deviance practitioners believe that the knowledge and ability
to solve a problem lies inside a community, and that challenges the traditional role of experts. While social change experts usually make a living
discerning community deficits, and then implementing outside solutions
to change them, in the PD approach, the role of experts is framed differently. The expert's role is to help the community find the positive deviants,
identify their uncommon but effective practices, and then to design a community intervention to make them visible and actionable.

In PD, change is led by those in the target group who present the *social proof* to their peers. Social proof is a psychological phenomenon in
which people come to believe that they can adopt a different practice because they discover people like them, in their own communities, using the
practice. The perception is that if others are doing something, it makes
sense to do it too. As the PD behaviors are already in practice, the solutions

can be implemented without delay or access to outside resources. Further, the benefits can be sustained over time.

Six months after the Sternins arrival in Vietnam, a beaming Mr. Nuu from the Vietnamese Ministry of Foreign Affairs handed them their renewed visa. They would end up living in Vietnam for six years.

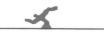

Pittsburgh, Pennsylvania, November 2004

In Jerry Sternin's words, "it is easier to act your way into a new way of thinking than to think your way into a new way of acting."

On a chilly November evening, Jon Lloyd, a retired general and vascular surgeon, was browsing the web site of the Plexus Institute in New Jersey and he came across an article published in the *Fast Company* magazine. The electronic article had *Vietnam* in its title, and it caught Lloyd's eye. In 1970-71, during the Vietnam War, he had served as a surgeon in the 3rd Field Army Hospital in Saigon. During his time in Vietnam, Lloyd fell in love with Vietnam and its people, including their hopes and aspirations, and their undoubting resilience.

The *Fast Company* article dealt with the resilience of Vietnam's poor people, who had found a way to combat childhood malnutrition using Positive Deviance.

"The article was like a ball of hot fire on my computer screen," Lloyd recalled. "It was the first time I heard about Positive Deviance. PD advocated local solutions—solutions that were owned by the people, not imported in by outside experts."

As the MRSA Prevention Coordinator assigned to the Office of the Chief of Staff at VA Pittsburgh Healthcare System (VAPHS), Lloyd was challenged by the limited outcomes gained using the Toyota Production System (TPS), an industrial, error-fixing approach to reducing health care-acquired infections (HAIs). He remembers: "In light of our TPS experience, I was looking—rather searching—for other approaches to combat MRSA infections—approaches that were more people-driven, sustainable, and not as resource intensive."

Intrigued by PD, Lloyd called the Positive Deviance Initiative and left a message.

Monique Sternin returned from overseas travel and returned the call several days later.

To his pleasant surprise, she told him that Waterbury Hospital in Connecticut had recently approached the Sternins to explore the possibility of using PD to address some of their intractable problems—complying with hand hygiene protocols to reduce infections, medication reconciliation at the time of patient discharge, and other patient safety issues. Lloyd learned that the Sternins had visited Waterbury Hospital and that the first application of a PD process in a U.S. health care facility seemed to be taking root.

The Waterbury Experiment: Deflecting a Health Care Boomerang

The PD enthusiasts at Waterbury Hospital were supported by CEO John Tobin and led by a dynamic nephrologist, Tony Cusano, who was also on the faculty of Yale Medical School. John Tobin had met Jerry Sternin in a workshop on health care quality and complexity science in June 2004 in Durham, New Hampshire, sponsored by Plexus Institute and the Harvard University Program for Health Systems Improvement. Tobin had returned to Waterbury intrigued about the application of the Positive Deviance approach for hand-hygiene compliance.

Tobin invited the Sternins to Waterbury to do a presentation on Positive Deviance later that year, and a core group of self-selected people, led by Cusano, coalesced around applying Positive Deviance to address an intractable problem. After much deliberation and consultation with the Sternins, Cusano's team decided to focus their PD efforts on medication reconciliation—patient adherence to medication regimes follow-

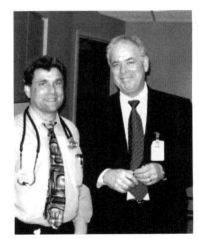

Nephrologist Tony Cusano and CEO John Tobin, PD enthusiasts at Waterbury Hospital

ing discharge from the hospital. Several factors are considered responsible for low compliance: poor communication, linguistic and cultural barriers, and lack of insurance covering prescriptions. When discharged patients don't take prescribed medicines, or take them incorrectly, their chances of another hospitalization escalate. That can lead to a downward spiral of more illness, more expense, more drugs, and more mistakes with prescribed medications.

As part of the PD discovery process, Cusano encouraged nurses, residents, and other hospital staff to make phone calls to discharged patients to gain firsthand feedback about how medications were being taken. He relied on his personal relationships with Waterbury staff members to get the process of making calls underway, and then encouraged the call-makers to enlist others in their personal network to do the same. This personal discovery of reconciliation problems fanning outward was crucial as it led other nurses, doctors, and residents to call more and more patients. As the network of callers expanded, more and more staff became aware of the widespread medication reconciliation problem. A critical mass of Waterbury staff was now engaged in the PD approach. Many more were intrigued. And several were skeptical, of course.

Several people at Waterbury described the phone calls as defining moments in the PD process. Magali Milfort, an advanced practice nurse, recalls that when she was asked if she would help collect data on medical reconciliation, she thought: "another thing I have to do…" Milfort hadn't seen Jerry Sternin's presentation at Waterbury's Grand Rounds and didn't know much about PD. After speaking with the first few patients in their homes however, she experienced what she called a huge "wake up call."

Milfort and several other nurses she subsequently enlisted to make calls described being shocked at what they discovered in their conversations with patients. Some patients had medications listed on their discharge sheets that weren't listed in their charts. Other patients had the correct list, but were not taking the medications because they could not find them at their local pharmacy, or they were too expensive. Nurses found the use of Latin abbreviations on discharge sheets was extremely confusing for patients. One nurse with 20 years experience was taken aback by that because, Latin or not, the information was clearly written.

To hospital staff, "Q.I.D" means *four times a day*, "B.I.D." is *two times a day* and "Q.H.S." means *take the medication at bedtime*. Some patients interpreted those directions to mean *every four hours* or *every two hours*. Many of the problems discovered in the phone calls were out of the control of hospital staff: patients' lack of adequate insurance coverage for prescription drugs, or no insurance at all, self-rationing of expensive medications to make them last longer, prioritizing the purchase of some meds over others when all meds prescribed needed to be taken together, and patients stopping meds because they felt better.

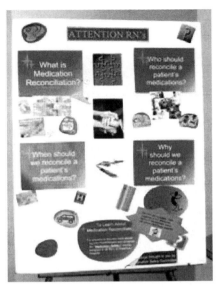

A poster of the complex medication reconciliation information flows at Waterbury reminds staff of ways to help patients comply

One big problem of medication overdosing was caused by the common practice of doctors writing: "resume all meds" on patient discharge sheets. A patient who had been taking one drug for high cholesterol before admission might be prescribed a similar drug during their hospitalization. Nurses who called patients at home would ask: "Are you taking the proper medications for your cholesterol?" To which the unwitting patient, happy to have received a call from the hospital, would reply: "Oh yes, I've been faithfully taking both my cholesterol drugs every day." At the time of discharge, the patient clearly did not grasp that the cholesterol drug administered temporarily during the hospital stay was to be discontinued, and that the pre-admission medication regimen was to be resumed.

At all hospitals, some patients are readmitted because of medication errors or non-adherence to medication plans after discharge. The phone contacts made by doctors, residents and nurses in fall of 2004 disclosed that 60 per cent of the discharged patients interviewed were not taking their medicines correctly. This shocking realization got people at Waterbury talking to one another about how to improve the process. As staff began discussions, they learned how some staff members were doing things differently, and having success.

Hospitalist Jay Kenkare recalls being told by a senior resident "a good discharge takes as long as an admission." Several nurses at Waterbury were indeed taking extra time to prepare their patients for discharge. "Deviant" nurses were putting Latin abbreviations into laymen's terms for patients, creating calendars to facilitate adherence to complex medical regimens like steroid tapering, and requesting that a family member be present while giving instructions to patients, to have an extra set of ears and eyes to increase comprehension. This practice was especially important when the patient was not a native English speaker. Phone calls to non-English speaking households revealed that patients who had said "yes, yes" when being asked if they understood instructions at discharge were in fact just eager to go home and hadn't understood a word of what had been said.

The phone calls also revealed that patients who were following their medication regimens as prescribed (the PD patients) were more likely to have received, at the time of discharge, what staff members call "the green sheet." Interestingly, this green sheet was a simple form and protocol that was developed by the Pharmacy and Therapeutics Committee at Waterbury, but only used 20 per cent of the time. However, as PD patients told more and more callers about the value of this tool used by some hospital staff, its use jumped to 75 per cent within a few months and with no new educational program or policy pronouncement.

Another technique used by nurses was to have patients write out their own medication list under nurse supervision. A helpful practice identified by patients was when the telephone numbers of the floor nurses' station were written on discharge sheets, in the event that patients had follow-up questions or needed clarification on dosages.

Doctors also had practices that differed from the norm. One doctor took pains to eliminate duplications caused by the "resume all meds" directive. Another went over new medications, one by one, with the patient as well as writing them on the discharge sheet, which would be issued, with repeated instructions, by the nurse.

After applying a cycle of PD processes with initial help from Jerry and Monique Sternin, Waterbury Hospital achieved a 66 per cent improvement in medication reconciliation. This significant increase resulted from a variety of positive deviant medication communication practices uncovered by staff. These improvements have been sustained for four years since the completion of the PD cycle with no further intervention.

VAPHS and MRSA: "Experts Right Under Our Noses"

Waterbury Hospital's pioneering foray into PD meant that Lloyd and the Sternins had much to talk about. After all, the lack of adherence to full courses of antibiotics has contributed to the emergence of deadly MRSA strains. Also, both MRSA control and medication reconciliation were closely aligned with patient safety issues and quality of care outcomes. A date was agreed upon in March 2005 for the Sternins to visit Pittsburgh.

Before the Sternins' visit, Lloyd shared the *Fast Company* article with VAPHS' Chief of Staff Rajiv Jain, who was intrigued: "PD seemed to overcome the two concerns I had with TPS—resources and ownership. PD was resource neutral. And it was premised on involvement of everyone." Jain convinced other members of VAPHS' senior leadership team that there was little to lose in trying this novel approach to address the MRSA problem.

In March 2005, Jerry Sternin did two workshops on PD in Pittsburgh. Representatives from local hospitals were invited. The VAPHS' two major facilities were represented. They were determined to tackle MRSA from a different direction.

In July 2005, Jerry and Monique Sternin returned to Pittsburgh do a follow-up workshop and consult with the VAPHS staff. They infused new energy, providing wind for VAPHS' expanding PD sails.

Endnotes

1. Kendra Cherry, "Selected Quotations by Psychologist Kurt Lewin." http://psychology.about.com/od/psychologyquotes/a/lewinquotes.htm (accessed 6-16-10).

2. M. Zeitlin, H. Ghassemi, M Mansour, *Positive deviance in child nutrition.* (New York: UN University Press 1990); Monique Sternin and the late Jerry Sternin in personal conversation and recorded interviews with Arvind Singhal in 2008 and 2009.

3. U. Mackintosh, D. Marsh, D. Schroeder, "Sustained positive deviant child care practices and their effects on child growth in Viet Nam," *Food and Nutrition Bulletin* 2002, Vol.23, No 4, (supplement) The United Nations University.

4. Anthony Cusano, "Positive Deviance: A New Process for Improving Professional Performance for Quality and Safety in the Health Care Setting," Waterbury Hospital, Waterbury, CT, (unpublished paper 2006).

5. Anthony Cusano, MD, in personal interview with Arvind Singhal, 5-29-09.

Chapter 3
Complex Problems, Complex Processes and Complexity Science
by Curt Lindberg

We live in a world that is becoming increasingly complex. Unfortunately, our style of thinking rarely matches this complexity.

— Gareth Morgan, Images of Organization

In the story about Positive Deviance told in the preceding chapter we learned of Vietnam villages that over the course of many years developed norms and habits, sustained through everyday conversations, about what were considered appropriate nutrition and feeding practices for young children. A consequence of these conversations and habits was a malnutrition rate of 64 per cent.

In many ways a similar story can be told about the scourge of MRSA in the United States. Both childhood malnutrition and infection prevention are complex problems defined by history, culture and social norms. They are not readily altered by technical fixes. Both affect the lives and health of countless community members. Like the previously unexamined nutrition practices in Vietnam, both good and bad practices around infection prevention—hand washing, antibiotic prescribing, isolation precautions, screening for MRSA, environmental cleaning—are shaped and sustained through routine interactions among health care workers. Consequences include the emergence of antibiotic resistance, transmission of antibiotic resistant bacterium in health care organizations, and high infection rates.

Fortunately for millions of children in Vietnam and patients in hospitals across North and South America, Jerry and Monique Sternin focused their attention on those few in the community—the positive deviants—who were doing things differently, not following unexamined conventional norms and practices. The Sternins realized these positive deviants held some keys to better health. From their broad international development experience the Sternins brought some of their hard-won lessons to their work in Vietnam and the development of PD as novel approach to social and behavioral change. They came to believe that:

- There is more expertise within a community than is generally recognized.

- Plans that emerge from within a community are more likely to be used and sustained than plans imposed from the outside.

- Relationships built through widespread community engagement in change efforts provide strong networks for the spread of good ideas and practices.

- Conversations fostered by broad involvement generate good new ideas.

- Diversity and difference are allies when you seek change.

- Practice of new behaviors, especially when married with information on results, supports change and learning.

As the Sternins were doing their pioneering work in Vietnam, some remarkably similar conclusions were being reached by pioneering scientists studying such seemingly disparate systems as insect colonies, the human brain, economies, forests, and families. Their scholarship has given rise to the young science of complexity, a science that seeks explanations for how change and order emerge in systems to all types. Stephen Hawking and

Edward O. Wilson have called it the science of the twenty-first Discoveries from this new discipline are being tapped to stimu... provements in health care by:

- Advancing management practice;[2]

- Examining factors that influence health care quality;[3]

- Informing nursing education;[4]

- Providing new insights into physiologic patterns in health and disease;[5]

- Increasing understanding of dynamics in health care organizations.[6]

Discoveries in complexity science provide a theoretical foundation for Positive Deviance and for understanding the nature of complex problems like the emergence of antibiotic resistance and childhood malnutrition.

Interacting Agents, Self-Organization and Emergence

Complex systems—like patients, communities, health care organizations, and MRSA—are comprised of interdependent agents—like organs in the body, community residents, health care workers, and cells—that interact with each other and the environment to create *emergent outcomes*. Examples of emergent outcomes include childhood malnutrition, resistance to antibiotics in bacteria, and health care-associated MRSA infection rates in hospitals. These outcomes emerge from a process scientists call *self-organization*. This term is meant to convey two points: that no one can control the emergent outcomes of a process driven by interactions among constantly changing agents; and, because of this complexity, no one can predict with certainty the future behavior and emergent outcomes of these systems. Surprises can arise at any time. Consider these points in light of such phenomena as stock market behavior, innovations like the internet, the emergence of life on earth, climate change, and behavior of bacteria. In an article aptly titled "Forever unprepared—the predictable unpredictability of pathogens," Sepkowitz wrote in *The New England Journal of Medicine*, "Nothing microbes do, whether under the duress imposed by antimicrobials, or from some less evident pressure, should surprise us. It's their world; we only live in it."[7]

Staphylococcus aureus, interacting with other bacteria, with antibiotics prescribed by health care professionals, and with patients, suddenly becomes resistant to penicillin and later an increasing array of antibiotics. Then a new strain of MRSA—community-associated MRSA—arrives on the scene, a development not foreseen by infectious disease experts.[8] In a similar fashion health care-associated MRSA rates in hospitals are a con-

Of Fireflies and Bridges, and Human Hands, Hearts and Feet: The Mysterious Rhythms of Synchrony

"All around us we see magnificent structures—galaxies, cells, ecosystems, human beings—that have somehow managed to assemble themselves." The mathematician Steven Strogatz has studied synchrony for decades, and he makes that intriguing observation in the first chapter of his book *Sync.* He calls synchrony "one of the most pervasive drives in the universe," one that extends from the subatomic to the cosmic, and "uses every communication channel that nature has invented."[1]

Scientists have observed synchrony near the rivers of Thailand and Malaysia where thousands of fireflies blink on and off in a steady rhythm and in unison. As Strogatz explains it, in a crowd of flashing fireflies, "every one is sending and receiving signals, shifting the rhythms of others and being shifted by them in return." In humans, it's the synchronization of cells that keeps our hearts working. A cluster

of thousands of cells generates the electrical rhythm that keeps the rest of the heart beating. These pacemaker cells, Strogatz explains, keep oscillating automatically, even in a Petri dish. And there are no maestro cells directing the others. The cellular collective coordinates individual action in a democratic way.[2]

Strogatz also tells the story of Christiaan Huygens, a Dutch physicist who invented the pendulum clock, which was far more accurate than any other time piece of its era. In 1665 Huygens discovered that the pendulums of two differently set clocks would begin oscillating together within half an hour. He had discovered *inanimate sync,* which Strogatz calls "the granddaddy of all complex systems." Planets and molecules seem to organize themselves in the same way.[3]

Scientists have studied many forms of human synchrony. Women who live together in dormitories and homes tend to have synchronized menstrual cycles, and researchers found that in proximity with one another, nonverbal communication happens through pheromones in sweat. Runners sometimes fall into harmony.

sequence of patterns of daily infection prevention practices (good and bad) of hospital staff, medical procedures, antibiotic usage, and interactions with the bacteria and patients themselves. They are also a consequence of how we think about organizations and change.

Conventional perspectives of organizations assume they operate like machines, like Newton's "clockwork" universe. Like watchmakers, managers and experts are organizational mechanics who fix things and expect repairs to work as intended. We give titles to these people like chief *exec-*

Sometimes living and inanimate things can fall into harmony. In June 2000, the Millennium Bridge was opened with great fanfare. It was an elegant new walkway over the Thames River, and the Queen presided as pedestrians began to cross. Suddenly the bridge started to sway from side to side. It was closed shortly thereafter for fear of some serious design or material defect.[4]

What actually happened was that pedestrians had been resonating with the bridge, and inadvertently amplified its movements. They unconsciously synchronized their steps as they walked; the more they did, the more the bridge wobbled, and the more it wobbled, the more they adjusted their steps. Strogatz called it the "unintended human synchrony caused by positive feedback." Strogatz and fellow mathematicians found that the bridge was steady with 150 people on it, but with 160 walkers, a threshold was crossed, and the structural wobbling and crowd synchronization emerged together.[5]

Researchers have observed self-organization in audience applause and in such visually dramatic examples as when crowds at sports events do "the wave."

Some crowd behavior, the adoption of fads and crazes, and movements of financial markets and highway traffic may also have to do with synchronicity. People like to sing and dance together. Strogatz, a leading scholar of the mathematical basis for self-organization, thinks deeper understanding of sync could revolutionize our views of all sorts of phenomena ranging from the origins of life to our understanding human behavior.

Notes

1. Steven Strogatz, *Sync: The Emerging Science of Spontaneous Order*, (New York: Hyperion Books, 2003), 1-2.

2. Ibid, 12-15.

3. Ibid, 104-8.

4. BBC News, Millennial Bridge, "Watch the Bridge Wobble." http://news.bbc.co.uk/hi/english/stati c/in_depth/uk/2000/millennium_brid ge/default.stm (accessed 6-04-10).

5. *Science Daily*, "Explaining Why the Millennium Bridge Wobbled." http://www.sciencedaily.com/release s/2005/11/051103080801.htm (accessed 6-10-10).

utive officers, chief *operating* officers, and infection *control* practitioners. Watchmakers change a gear or adjust a spring and the watch keeps time again. Health care managers and infection control experts gather the best evidence, write policies and conduct extensive education programs for staff on the new procedures and understandably expect adherence to the new standards. Unfortunately, life in an organization is generally not this simple and straightforward (and bacteria do not read hospital policies).

Simple, Complicated and Complex

A framework that can help us make sense of traditional management thinking in light of developments in complexity science and new change processes such as Positive Deviance was developed by Glouberman and Zimmerman.[9] It suggests that problems can be thought of as *simple, complicated* or *complex*. The example they provide of a *simple* challenge is baking a cake. Follow the recipe, and the likely outcome is a cake. There are clear connections between cause and effect: ingredients, the correct baking time and a cake emerges from the oven. Going to the moon is much more challenging than baking a cake. In the Gouberman-Zimmerman framework this challenge is *complicated*. Success requires great scientific expertise, a high degree of coordination and sophisticated communication systems. When these are in place one can reasonably predict the outcome and, with practice, the outcomes generally improve over time.

Raising a child (think teenager) is *complex*. The outcome is unpredictable. There are some books written by experts and there are child development specialists, but following the guidance provided does not guarantee success. Here is where insights from complexity science can be most helpful. Each child is unique and changes in response to a variety of forces and interactions that cannot be controlled. A maturing child has increasing discretion. Shaping the development of a child is fundamentally done through relationships and interactions, and the interactions affect not only the child but parents, friends and teachers.

Frances Westley, Brenda Zimmerman and Michael Paton argue that "successful innovation combines all three problems—simple, complicated and complex—but the least understood is complex. And yet, complexity is the most fundamental level when we try to understand how social innovations occur."[10]

The Surprising Influence of Interactions

Like raising a child, future changes in MRSA and hospital infection rates can neither be directly controlled nor predicted; at its core, the problem is complex. Complexity science suggests these changes will depend heavily on alterations in interactions in these systems. In human systems, complexity scientists suggest there are several factors that exert a strong influence on self-organization: information flow; the number and nature of interactions; the diversity of agents; and shifts in power differentials.[11] Using these parameters, health care researchers are beginning to demonstrate that quality of patient care as an emergent outcome is related to "positive local interaction patterns" where health care workers effectively exchange "new information, develop high-quality relationships, and foster cognitive diversity in decision making."[12]

Future changes in MRSA and hospital infection rates can neither be directly controlled nor predicted; at its core, the problem is complex.

While this body of research developed independently of the work by the Sternins, it is clear the PD process exploits these four factors. Using PD actively invokes diversity by engaging people not typically involved in guiding improvement efforts (the Sternins call them "unusual suspects") and uncovering deviant (read different) practices and strategies. New connections are developed by inviting an ever-widening number of people to join in shaping the process; power and decision-making are shared; participants are constantly asking "Who else should be here?" Those engaged in PD-informed efforts build new relationships and share new information through a broadening network of conversations.

As illustrated in the Vietnam story and the work of hospitals to prevent the spread of infections, matching the complexity of the intervention with the complexity of the problem and influencing the self-organizing process can lead to improvements in emergent outcomes: fewer malnourished children and fewer patients afflicted by infections.

We have also witnessed the spread of a novel social and behavioral change process from a few villages in Vietnam to many other communities and organizations around the world. This dynamic, a small action trigger-

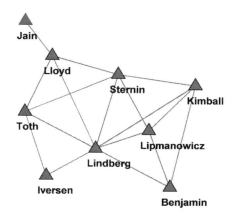

Network of individuals who, in 2005, initially explored
the application of PD for MRSA prevention
(Network maps courtesy of Chris Black and June Holley)

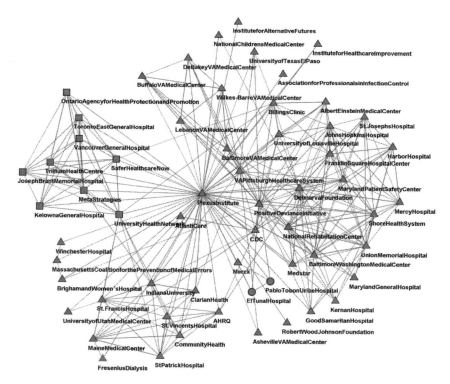

Network of organizations in 2010
dedicated to using PD to prevent health care-associated infections

ing a large change, is another universal feature of complex systems. Scientists call this *nonlinearity*. It was first recognized by M.I.T. meteorologist Edward Lorenz in his study of weather forecasting and popularized in his famous 1982 talk "Predictability: does the flap of a butterfly's wings in Brazil set off a tornado in Texas?"[13] In the story of the application of PD in health care one small change—a conversation that took place among nine individuals in 2005—led to an ever-expanding network of health care organization using Positive Deviance to prevent health care-associated infections. In 2010, this network numbered more than fifty-nine institutions and thousands of people across the U.S., South America and Canada. The small change to large change dynamic is evident in the two network maps on the previous page.

Each of the stories about the use of Positive Deviance in hospitals featured in the following chapters will be followed by brief editor reflections. Through this vehicle we hope to highlight key principles of PD and complexity science, give readers a good sense for the fullness of the PD process, and demonstrate how it was adapted to work in a variety of different hospital cultures.

Endnotes

1. G. Chui, "Unified theory is getting closer, Hawking predicts," *San Jose Mercury News,* 2000, section A; R. Lindberg, and D. Hutchens, "Edward O. Wilson Speaks on Complexity," *Emerging* 2002, January/February, 5-9.

2. R. Anderson, L. Issel, R. McDaniel, "Nursing homes as complex adaptive systems: relationship between management practice and resident outcomes," *Nursing Research* vol. 62, no. 1, 2003, 12-21; R. Stacey, *Complexity and Creativity in Organizations,* (San Francisco: Berrett-Kohler, 1996); R. Stacey, *Strategic Management and Organisational Dynamics: The Challenge of Complexity to Ways of Thinking About Organisations,* 5th edition, (London: Pearson Education, 2007); R. McDaniel, R. and D. Driebe, "Complexity science and health care management," in *Advances in health care management,* vol. 2, 2001; J. Blair, M. Fottler, and G. Savage, eds., JAI Press, Stamford, 11-36; Zimmerman, B., Lindberg, C. and Plsek, P. *Edgeware: Insights from Complexity Science for Health Care Leaders,* (Irving, TX: VHA Inc., 1998).

3. R. Anderson and R. McDaniel, "Taking complexity science seriously: new research, new methods," in *On the Edge: Nursing in the Age of Complexity,* C. Lindberg, S. Nash, and C. Lindberg, eds. (Bordentown, NJ: PlexusPress, 2008) 73-95. Committee on Quality of Health Care in America, Institute of Medicine, *Crossing the Quality Chasm, A New Health System for the 21st Century,* (Washington, DC: National Academy Press, 2001); Anderson, "Nursing Homes as Complex Adaptive Systems."

4. Lindberg, *On the Edge, Nursing in the Age of Complexity.*

5. A. Goldberger, "Fractal variability versus pathologic periodicity: complexity loss and stereotypy in disease, *Perspectives in Biology and Medicine*, vol. 40, no. 4, 1997, 543-561; B. West, "A physicist looks at physiology," in Lindberg, *On the Edge: Nursing in the Age of Complexity*, 97-123; B. West, *Where Medicine Went Wrong: Rediscovering the Path to Complexity,* (Singapore: World Scientific, 2006).

6. B. Zimmerman, *Edgeware;* McDaniel, "Complexity science and health care management"; W. Miller, et al, "Practice jazz: understanding variation in family practice using complexity science," *The Journal of Family Practice*, vol. 50, no. 10, 2001, 872-878.

7. K. Sepkowitz, "Forever unprepared—the predictable unpredictability of pathogens," *The New England Journal of Medicine*, vol. 361, no. 2, 2009, 120-121.

8. Sepkowitz, "Forever unprepared."

9. S. Glouberman and B. Zimmerman, "Complicated and complex systems: what would successful reform of Medicare look like," in *Health Care Services and the Process of Change*, P. Forest, T. McKintosh and G. Marchilden, eds., (Toronto: University of Toronto Press, 2004).

10. F. Westley, B. Zimmerman, B. and M. Patton, M., *Getting to Maybe: How the World is Changed,* (Toronto: Random House Canada, 2006), 10.

11. S. Kauffman, *At Home in the Universe: The Search for the Laws of Self-Organization,* (New York: Oxford University Press, 1995); J. Holland, *Emergence: From Chaos to Order,* (Cambridge, MA: Perseus Books, 1998); R. Stacey, *Strategic Management and Organisational Dynamics: The Challenge of Complexity to Ways of Thinking About Organizations*, 5th edition, (London: Pearson Education, 2007).

12. Anderson and McDaniel, "Taking complexity science seriously," 1986.

13. E. Lorenz, *The Essence of Chaos,* (Seattle: University of Washington Press, 1993).

Chapter 4
Small Solutions and Big Rewards: MRSA Prevention at the Pittsburgh Veterans Hospitals
by Arvind Singhal and Karen Greiner

Serendipitous discoveries are always made by people in a particular frame of mind, people who are focused and alert because they are searching for something. They just happen to find something else.

— Steven Strogatz, *Sync*

How can you combat a hearty bacterium that can survive for weeks on any surface anywhere in the hospital? At the VA Pittsburgh Healthcare System (VAPHS) people working on the problem concluded that they couldn't control a bug that anyone can transmit unless they invited everyone from all parts of the system to join the fight.

This culture of invitation is what made a member of the housekeeping staff feel comfortable enough to teach "a thing or two" about hygiene to the rest of the unit, explained Cheryl Creen, MRSA coordinator at VAHPS'

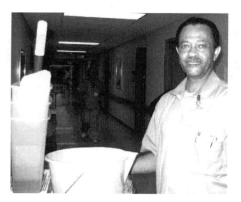

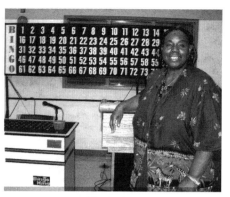

Housekeeping staff member
Edward Yates

Tanis Smith, the zapper

Heinz long-term care facility. One day, she said, some staff members were talking about cleaning the room of a patient with C-diff (*Clostridium diffi-cile*) "and Eddie Yates, from housekeeping, stepped forward and said 'alcohol won't work on spores of C-diff. We have to use Clorox'." In hospitals where communication typically happens along departmental lines according to the traditional hierarchy, this was an important shift.

Tanis Smith is a recreational therapist who supervises the evening Bingo game. After the game is over, and the reusable bingo cards put away, Smith walks down the aisle, squirting anti-bacterial foam into the patients' open palms, calling: "Get your zap and get your snack." When a veteran with only one arm, a regular at the Bingo session, holds out his hand, she squirts a dab of foam on to her palms, washing his hand with hers.

Some veterans who have faced danger on the battlefield tend to scoff at germs, but, according to Smith, even the toughest can be felled by infection. "Interestingly, once a few veterans begin to practice hand hygiene in public, there is increasing pressure on others to comply," Smith observed.

Just How Dangerous Are These MRSA Bacteria?

At the VAPHS, MRSA Coordinator Heidi Walker used macaroni to address this question. She loaded 21 bags of macaroni onto a gurney along with hand foam dispensers, gloves, gowns, and nasal swabs. As a curious audience of patients, nurses, doctors, and other staff persons listened to

Walker's primer on MRSA and health care-associated infections (HAIs), she cracked open a bag, scooped up a handful of macaroni, and dropped the uncooked pieces into an empty plastic bowl one by one. Each piece, she said, represented a human life lost as a result of HAIs. She then pointed to the macaroni bags on the gurney—they contained a total of 100,000 pieces—the total number of lives lost each year to HAIs in U.S. hospitals.

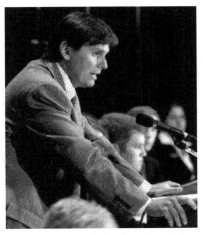

John Jernigan, MD, infectious disease specialist, CDC

"Heidi's demonstration had a strong emotional effect on the audience," said Jon Lloyd, MD, a retired general and vascular surgeon and Plexus Institute's Senior Clinical Advisor, who served between 2004 to 2007 as the Coordinator of MRSA Prevention for VAPHS. Walker used sight and sound in a startling demonstration that brought statistics to life.

Welcome Serendipity

The VAPHS got involved in MRSA prevention serendipitously. John Jernigan, MD, is a CDC expert in the epidemiology of health care-associated infections and presently CDC's deputy chief, Prevention and Response Branch, Division of Healthcare Quality Promotion. In 2001 he began to collaborate with the Pittsburgh Regional Health Initiative (PRHI) on "zero goals," an initiative to eliminate hospital-acquired infections and medication errors. VAPHS agreed to carry out CDC's pilot MRSA prevention initiative in its surgical ward and intensive care unit.

TPS, Kaizen by Reducing Errors and Defects

The framework for the CDC-PRHI-VAPHS MRSA prevention collaboration was derived from the principles of the Toyota Production System (TPS). Kaizen is a Japanese term that refers to a philosophy of continuous

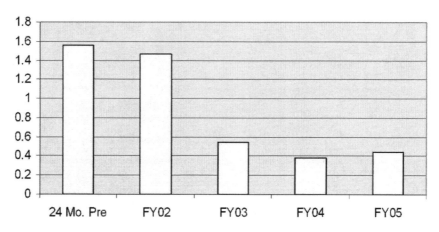

MRSA Infections/1000 BDOC - Surgical Ward

A 70 per cent drop in MRSA infection rates on Unit 4W after TPS was implemented (BDOC indicates Bed-Days of Care)

improvement in all work processes. The theory was that processes that helped reduce mistakes and defects on production shop floors all over the world could help reduce errors that jeopardized patient safety. Peter Perreiah, formerly Production System Manager at Alcoa, served as team leader of the MRSA prevention initiative in the surgical ward, located in 4 West of the VAPHS' University Drive facility. A month later, staff nurse Ellesha McCray joined Perreiah on the TPS team.

McCray and Perreiah gathered baseline data by observing staff-patient encounters in 4 West. After talking with many staff members, they concluded that the staff perception was that "MRSA infections were primarily because of overuse of antibiotics, and not because of what *they* did or did not do."

Management of supplies was a problem. The nurses would don gowns or gloves only if they were easily accessible and the stock was continually replenished. However, accountability was diffused: for instance, it was unclear who was responsible for keeping supplies in stock. "TPS is about standardization," explained McCray. "But, in a hospital, we are talking about people; you can't standardize everything. So you standardize what you can."

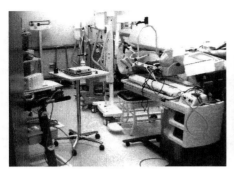 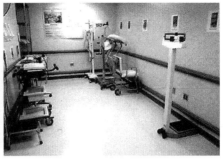

Equipment room on 4 West pre-TPS Equipment room on 4 West post-TPS

During the three years (from 2001 to 2004) that Perreiah and McCray were TPS team leaders MRSA infections dropped in the 4 West surgical ward by a whopping 70 per cent.

TPS helped put several new systems in place, some of which spread system-wide at VAPHS. Before TPS for instance, staff members at 4 West found it hard to access machines such as the crash cart in the equipment room. The room was cluttered and cords were often entangled.

Post-TPS, each piece of equipment was stored in a designated place—labeled in big bold letters and with a visual image to avoid any confusion.

Before TPS, the supply room was a similar mess. Often, syringes, catheters, or aerosol chambers were inaccessible or haphazardly stored. The inventories were often a mystery; ordering was inefficient and erratic. An item might not be reordered until sometime realized the supply was gone. Post-TPS, each item was neatly labeled, and stored by type and function in color-coded bins.

VAPHS' Chief of Staff Rajiv Jain, MD, noted that hospital management was "very pleased" with the steep decline in MRSA infection rates on 4 West, and in late 2003, expanded TPS to University Drive's surgical intensive care unit (SICU). MRSA infection rates at SICU dropped by an impressive 70 per cent over the next two years.

By mid-2005, VAPHS executives wanted to expand the MRSA prevention program beyond the two units on University Drive. Jain explained: "TPS was effective but it had two shortcomings. First, TPS required additional resources—and we were not in a position to hire another 10 to 12 Peter Perreiahs and Ellesha McCrays for our other units. It was slow and

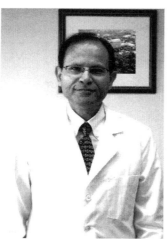

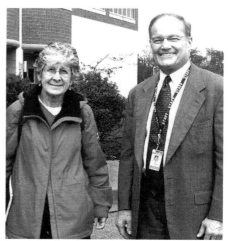

Dr. Rajiv Jain, chief of staff, VAPHS

Jon Lloyd (R) with Monique Sternin of the Positive Deviance Initiative at VAPHS' Heinz facility

expensive. Second, I got the sense that the program had the appearance of being run by the team leaders."

As the MRSA Prevention Coordinator, Jon Lloyd was challenged by the limited outcomes offered by the TPS approach. TPS' impact on the successful MRSA control effort on the 4 West and the SICU at University Drive had not spread through the 13 units at VAPHS. "In light of our TPS experience, I was looking—rather searching—for other approaches to combat MRSA; approaches that were more people-driven, sustainable, and not as resource intensive," Lloyd said.

Serendipitously, in November, 2004, when Lloyd was browsing the web site of Plexus Institute, he read an article in *Fast Company* magazine about PD used to fight childhood malnutrition in Vietnam. In March, 2005, Jerry and Monique Sternin, the founders of the Positive Deviance Initiative, conducted two workshops on the PD process in Pittsburgh. Some 50 representatives from 10 Pittsburgh area hospitals attended. The VAPHS' two major facilities—University Drive, an acute care facility, and the Heinz long-term care facility—were represented.

Lloyd remembers: "When Jerry Sternin arrived in Pittsburgh, given his previous work in Vietnam and other countries, I was ready to greet someone sporting a pony tail, faded jeans, worn out sandals, and beads. However, he seemed like a normal guy, sporting a jacket and a tie." Yet Lloyd remembered "many at VAPHS were skeptical that an approach that was effective to combat childhood malnutrition in Vietnam would hold relevance for MRSA control in a U.S. health care system."

For others, like Jain and Lloyd, the notion of amplifying "what works" in addition to fixing "what does not work" held promise.

As Lloyd noted: "The U.S. health care industry has been too focused, for too long, on fixing errors. Too preoccupied with making right what is wrong. Nurses and hospital staff have been bombarded with a litany of top-down expert-driven directives to fix a broken system. In this context, PD's focus on 'what works' was greeted with open arms." Referring to Tanis Smith's foamy zap before the snack in Heinz's bingo room, Lloyd emphasized, "The expertise to tackle MRSA is right under our noses. There are hundreds of experts here; the key is recognizing that the solutions to the problem exist among the staff and the patients."

"Nurses and hospital staff have been bombarded with a litany of top-down directives to fix a broken system. In this context, PD's focus on 'what works' was greeted with open arms."

In July 2005, Jerry and Monique returned to Pittsburgh do a follow-up PD workshop and consult with the VAPHS staff. They infused new energy, providing enthusiasm for expanding the PD work. A core group of PD champions began to emerge.

Expanding the Solution Space

Following the Sternins' July 2005 visit, dozens of focus group interviews involving staff from throughout the hospital—nurses, doctors, patients, custodians, van drivers, pastors, lab technicians—were conducted over several weeks at times most convenient to the staff to solicit all kinds of ideas for preventing MRSA. These discussions eventually were dubbed "Discovery and Action Dialogues" because of the action-oriented outcomes they yielded. Several walls of sticky yellow Post-it Notes captured diverse, staff-generated ideas on controlling MRSA. Out of these 50-plus dialogues, which engaged more than 500 staff members from all specialties and vocations at the VAPHS, hundreds of solutions were generated. These included recommendations to place foam dispensers in the recreation room, in the cafeteria, and in the library, where the likelihood of touching the same bingo cards, the same serving spoon, or the same newspaper is very high.

Ira Richmond, associate director for patient care services at VAPHS said, "The evolution of the PD program has been phenomenal in helping to support a model of what, in nursing, we call 'shared governance'—staff taking responsibility for MRSA prevention and control. And because the staff *owns* the solutions they propose, they comply with them."

"When the staff sees that a patient on their unit has converted from MRSA negative to MRSA positive, they put on their Sherlock Holmes hats to deduce how that transmission might have happened," Richmond said. "Then they develop an intervention to address the problem."

Joyce Ewing, the nurse manager of the SICU at University Drive facility said such deduction and problem solving often occur at the weekly MRSA briefings in VAPHS' acute and long-term care facility. The unit staff (including housekeepers, nurses, attending doctors) meets with MRSA coordinators and other administrative leaders to review their MRSA performance data, deduce reasons for any MRSA transmissions and the steps taken to reduce them. These recurring briefings provide an opportunity for the unit staff to also identify barriers to change, providing MRSA coordinators and administrators an opportunity to eliminate them. Their ideas and proposals signified the expanded range of solutions for MRSA prevention, control, and elimination at the VAPHS.

Glowing Germs

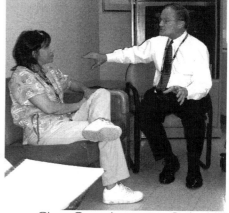

When Nurse Cathy Hill at Heinz's long-term care unit heard that the hospital staff was being encouraged to provide suggestions about how to combat MRSA, she was leery. Twelve years of nursing experience had taught her that MRSA was a formidable, invisible enemy, lurk-

Glow Germ innovator Cathy Hill
with Jon Lloyd

ing on curtains, light switches, gowns, handrails, and on the patients' skin and clothing.

Someone told her about a product that made germs glow. Hill searched the Internet and found Glo Germ, an invisible substance—available as liquid, gel, or powder—that glows when exposed to ultraviolet light. The Glo Germ arrived at Heinz just in time for her to arrange a stealth demonstration. The setting was perfect. In March 2006, VAPHS organized a day of MRSA stock-taking and results demonstration, and Hill smeared Glo Germ powder on the pens that attendees used to sign in. Around the corner, out of sight, was an ultraviolet light apparatus, awaiting the unsuspecting guinea pigs. As the day wore on, several scores of people were ushered to this apparatus.

When the staff sees that a patient on their unit has converted from MRSA negative to MRSA positive, they put on their Sherlock Holmes' hats to deduce how that transmission might have happened.

"People were shocked to see how the Glo Germ had unsuspectingly spread," Hill recalled. Under the UV light, the Glo Germ glowed on their hands and heads, shirts and skirts, glasses and watches, and on plates and cups. "It was everywhere…on everything they touched," she said.

MRSA's invisible cloak of transmission was now visible.

(In)Visible Signs

One of the visible signs of the VAPHS' efforts to combat MRSA is the alcohol hand hygiene dispensers lining its hallways; they are everywhere—in the recreation rooms, dining rooms, ceramic rooms, and the library. In the dementia unit, where such dispensers are a hazard, nurses have hand rub "holsters" on their belts or hand rub "necklaces"—miniature dispensers strung on a yarn. While hand rub dispensers are highly visible, there are hundreds of MRSA countermeasures that are below the radar, hidden from plain view.

Kathleen Risa's anti-MRSA trick is "the knuckle." Risa, who is now education coordinator, VHA MRSA Program Office, always pushes the elevator button with her knuckle, not a fingertip—which is likely a more potent vector of microbial transfer. There were several other anti-pathogen strategies: the "inside jacket gloving" technique in which the inside of a jacket is used to lock and unlock doors of toilet stalls; the "foot pedal flushing" to flush the toilet; and the "elbow side-arm swivel" to shut off the water faucet.

From Rock Logic to Water Logic

Edward De Bono describes two different types of thinking.[1] *Rock logic* is rock-like, hard and unyielding; something that sits on a surface and does not budge. *Water logic,* on the other hand, is water-like: soft and fluid. It spreads out and explores when flowing on a surface.

Hospitals are bastions of rock logic. Operating in a highly controlled regulatory environment, strict guidelines govern the practice of medicine. Processes are prioritized and protocol reigns supreme. Uncertainty and ambiguity are unwelcome and need to be vanquished. The metaphor of a "well-oiled machine" is valorized; each part should know what "is" and "should be." Clearly this rock logic is useful in the implementation of technical processes. However, it can be limiting.

Jennifer Scott, a nurse in Heinz's 2 South Unit, described a series of recent events on her floor that illustrate some shifts in thinking from rock to water logic. Scott credits the PD-inspired processes at Heinz for such a cultural shift.

A patient on Scott's floor was sinking rapidly and a "code red" alert went out on the hospital intercom. "The patient had 'alphabet soup'—all the germs one could possibly get," she said. "And I remember, outside the patient's room someone was playing the role of a sentry, dispensing gowns and gloves at the door. You couldn't get in unless you were properly gowned and gloved. There were people dashing in—doctors, nurses, nursing assistants, respiratory therapists, and others—from other floors. One of the doctors had 10 extra pairs of gloves in her pocket that she handed out to people as they came in."

While the patient's room was a beehive of activity, Scott remembers thinking: "What about the crash cart, the portable cart on which all the emergency supplies and resuscitation equipment was wheeled down? How is it cleaned? What happens to a monitor that has to be placed on an infected patient's bed just so that the cord could be plugged into the nearest electric outlet? Or what happens to the electric cord itself?"

Scott's acute awareness of how people and equipment move in an emergency led to her to pose questions inspired by water logic. Her thoughts focused not only on what is—the code red—but also on what *will be*: where do the crash cart and its equipment and supplies, go to *during* and *after* the cart's use?

"I'm thinking that sooner or later this screen is going to go if we keep cleaning it," she said, pointing to the EKG monitor sitting on the top shelf of the mobile cart.

After a pause, she continued: "What if we wrapped the screen in plastic separately? Then if we used the EKG monitor we could just change the plastic instead of cleaning the screen and everything else on the cart...."

At VAPHS new ideas, like water, continue to flow.

Cheryl's Relational Infrastructure

One of the first things you see when you enter Cheryl Creen's office is a typewritten sheet of paper on the bulletin board: "The question isn't who is going to let me, it's who is going to stop me."

As MRSA coordinator at Heinz, one of Creen's major duties is to follow up on ideas and suggestions offered by staff. "They need to know we're listening," she explained.

Creen often sticks her neck out to embody the "who is going to stop me" message that good ideas get implemented. Nonetheless, she acknowledges the constraints of the VA system, including keeping abreast of shifting government regulations. But, she adds, it's important that the staff know the regulations. This may mean having to explain "why a seemingly good idea can't be implemented—at least, not in the short term."

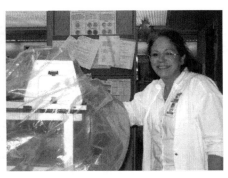
Nurse Jennifer Scott with the "clean" crash cart

British sociologist Anthony Giddens warned against the tendency to identify structure solely as constraint. Structure, according to Giddens, is both enabling and constraining.[2] The enormous structure that is the Veterans Administration operates within a necessary framework of guidelines, rules and regulations. Part of Creen's job is to create a space, within that structure, for her staff to think creatively. And, in Creen's world, everyone has something to contribute.

For example, at Heinz, a patient group was formed to harness the creative capacity of veterans themselves to combat MRSA. The idea of establishing this group was floated in one of the many "discovery dialogues" held by staff.

"Patients are not the problem. We could be part of the solution," noted Darryl, a veteran who acquired a MRSA infection at the VAPHS not knowing what it was, and faced four painful surgeries on his infected leg wound. "If one guy is contaminated, he can contaminate others." Darryl said he wished he had been able to inform a fellow veteran about the dangers of MRSA before he, too, ended up infected, lamenting, "If I could have gotten to him two days earlier…"

Darryl and his group created their own anti-MRSA brochure. The hospital-produced brochure is entitled "Resistant Bacteria: Methicillin Resistant Staphylococcus aureus and Vancomycin Resistant Enterococcus."

The title of the patient-produced brochure represents a different view: "Keeping America's Veterans Healthy—A Guide to MRSA—A simple way to shorten your stay."

Both brochures have a section on risk. Interestingly, the patient-produced brochure stresses that everyone who enters a hospital is at risk of *becoming a carrier*. The hospital-produced brochure notes that healthy people are at very little risk of *getting an infection* with resistant bacteria. Both statements are true but each is framed differently.

The patient-produced brochure exhorts veterans to become active in MRSA prevention. Lines on the last page of the brochure read: "Join in the effort to prevent its spread to other veterans. Ask a nurse how you can help." The difference in the patient and hospital-produced brochures illustrates how expanding the solution space to include patients provoked insightful perspective on MRSA prevention and control not considered before.

Further, the patient-produced brochure is credible with other patients. Trusting a fellow soldier, and covering each other's flank, is key to survival in a battlefield, and veterans at the VAPHS are expanding the application of these principles in another form of combat—with an invisible and dangerous enemy.

Display the Results for All to See

Through Glo Germ demonstrations, foam zaps after bingo, macaroni routines, and Discovery and Action Dialogues, a collective mindfulness about combating and eliminating MRSA is shaping up, especially at VAPHS' Heinz facility. Cheryl Creen, Candace Cunningham, and Jon Lloyd, VAPHS' MRSA commanders, worked hard to create feedback loops, so that experiences of one unit can be shared with other units, victories can be celebrated, and disappointments can be met with resolve.

Charts prominently displayed at all nursing stations at Heinz and University Drive provide the status of new MRSA infections and transmissions of the past week. During the weekly briefings, when the unit staff proudly announces: "no new MRSA infections during this past week," there are several rounds of applause.

Collective Mindfulness

Two years into the implementation of the PD MRSA initiative, many at VAPHS talk about the slow but perceptible culture change in the institution. For Cheryl Squier, the head infection control nurse at the VAPHS, the culture change was explained by "widespread ownership of the problem. The typical attitude in the past was: 'That's your department—you take care of it.' Today, MRSA is viewed as everyone's problem."

Robert Muder, MD, director of infection control, echoed Creen's sentiment: "I'm having more fun at this job and I'm also working harder—but now, instead of kicking down doors trying to get attention for infection control, front line staff are stepping up—at all levels, from housekeeping to the lab."

Ginny Rudy, VAPHS' nursing program leader, talked about the culture change at the VAPHS in terms of how infection control data is collected, shared, and acted upon. Ginny noted that the feedback staff receives about the regularly collected MRSA data, along with the opportunity they have to question and talk about what to do about it, has increased staff involvement: "When they see the data they see the difference their actions make."

Rudy illustrated her point. "About a year ago we had an in-house celebration about our 'victories' against MRSA and I personally invited all the lab technicians to join us. We showed them the poster-size infection charts that highlighted the reduced MRSA infection rates over time. Before this event, the lab technicians saw VAPHS' fight against MRSA as simply more work for them," she said. "But when they saw the prominently displayed MRSA control data—that is, the results of their own hard work—they realized the important role they were playing in this process. They seemed to suddenly understand that what they do makes a difference."

Making the Invisible Visible: Nightingale's Pioneering Coxcombs

In 1855 a young British nurse, Florence Nightingale, arrived in Scutari (in modern-day Istanbul), to care for British soldiers wounded in the Crimean War. Nightingale was appalled at the conditions in the Scutari hospital. Medicine was in short supply, hygiene and sanitation were neglected, and soldiers died en masse of infectious diseases. During Nightingale's

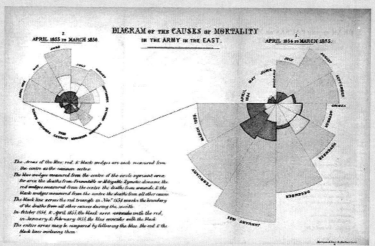

Nightingale's coxcomb depicting the seasonal rates of mortality among patients in the Scutari hospital. Each region shows the number of soldiers who died and the casues of their deaths. The right diagram depicts the mortality figures for each month from April 1854 to March 1855 before the sanitary procedures were implemented. The small black areas represent deaths due to wounds, the lighter colored areas represent deaths resulting from infectious diseases and other causes. The dramatic reductions in mortality rates from April, 1855 to March, 1856 are represented in the left diagram

Lloyd noted, "A true cultural transformation has occurred from within—with support from the leadership that demonstrated faith in its people—which manifests itself in a growing sense of ownership among staff and patients of the MRSA problem and their creation and implementation of hundreds of small solutions."

The top administrators at VAPHS repeatedly emphasized the importance of ensuring that the stories of staff member's contributions, however small, are told and celebrated.

Joyce Ewing recalled: "I was so thrilled by the precipitous decline in infection rates on the surgical intensive care unit over the past several years that I carried the printout in my pocket for *two weeks*. It's rare to get good

her first winter in Scutari, 4,077 soldiers died. To Nightingale's horror, ten times more soldiers died from illnesses, such as typhus, typhoid fever, cholera and dysentery, than from battle wounds.[1]

Six months after Nightingale's arrival the British government sent a sanitary commission to Scutari, flushing out the hospital sewers, improving lighting and ventilation, and laying out protocols for cleaning hospital equipment. Nightingale trained several dozen nurses in hygiene and sanitation, reorganizing patient care. Death rates dropped precipitously.[2]

During the Crimean War, Nightingale invented a visual mapping technique called the *coxcomb*, a modern circular histogram (also known as the rose diagram) to illustrate seasonal sources of patient mortality in her military hospital. She used this circular statistical representation and other novel statistical graphics to dramatize the appalling rates of death from preventable infections to Queen Victoria, Members of Parliament and civil servants, goading them to action.

Known the world-over as the Lady with the Little Lamp, few know that Nightingale was an unlikely candidate to pursue a career in nursing. Born in the lap of luxury (her parents' estate employed 70 gardeners), Nightingale horrified her parents by announcing her passion for nursing, which she saw as her divine calling. A nurse of nurses, Nightingale, who lived until age 90, was the second most famous British citizen, after Queen Victoria.

Notes

1. This section draws upon various sources, including: Absolute Astronomy, "Florence Nightingale: Facts, Discussion Forum. http://www.absoluteastronomy.com/topics/Florence_Nightingale; (accessed 6-17-10); Nancy Sokoloff, *Three Victorian Women Who Changed Their World*, London: Macmillan, 1982), and Cecil Woodham-Smith, *Florence Nightingale, 1820-1810*, (London: Penguin, 1955).

2. *Science News*, Math Trek: Florence Nightingale: Passionate Statistician. http://www.sciencenews.org/view/access/id/38939/title/jr_mtrek_nightingale (accessed 6-17-10).

news on this unit as we deal with the sickest patients." Then she added, "Once, I remember taking the graph out of my pocket with pride and showing it to my boss and saying, '*This* is what you pay me for'."

Clearly, hundreds of VAPHS staff members at all levels and in all units, and patients, are working together on hundreds of small solutions to prevent MRSA transmissions and associated infections.

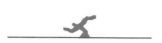

"I was so thrilled by the decline in infection rates that I carried the printout in my pocket for two weeks.
I took the graph out of my pocket with pride and showed it to my boss and said, 'This is what you pay me for.'"

Declining MRSA Rates at VAPHS

What evidence exists for declining MRSA rates at the VAPHS in aggregate terms, as well as in its two facilities—University Drive for acute care and Heinz for long-term care? How much of this decline may be attributed to the system-wide adoption of Positive Deviance practices—first at Heinz starting mid-2005, and then slowly at University Drive starting in 2006, where the TPS hangover may have been difficult for some to shake off. Jon Lloyd and Rajiv Jain provided the following responses to the above questions, based on the MRSA surveillance data at VAPHS.

Hospital-acquired surgical site MRSA infection rates declined by 50 per cent at VAPHS from July 2005 (when PD practices were implemented) to October, 2006.

Dramatic reductions in MRSA incidence occurred on 4 West and SICU prior to the introduction of PD, and since the introduction of PD in July 2005 the numbers of house-wide infections have declined even more precipitously.

Over the longer term, from 2005 (when the PD program was introduced) to 2009, MRSA infections dropped by up to 60 per cent according to Jain.

Jon Lloyd noted: "The true significance of this result is that while surgical site MRSA infection rates are declining at VAPHS, they have quintupled over the past decade nationally." Numbers aside, PD's contribution to declining MRSA infection rates at the VAPHS is noticeable in the level of staff engagement. Examples include the weekly unit-level MRSA briefings, and the generation and ownership of solutions to reduce MRSA, such as the "zap and snack" routine of Tanis Smith. Such qualitative outcomes synergistically contribute to MRSA prevention and control at the VAPHS, even if they are not directly countable. Many participants refer to increases in staff morale, which they believe *counts* significantly in reducing MRSA even if it may be hard to count in numerical terms.

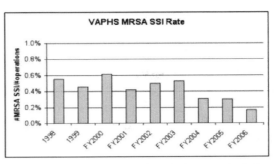

Declining surgical site MRSA infection rates at VAPHS

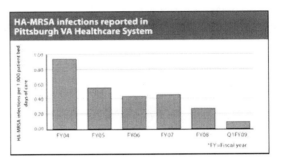

Long-term decline in MRSA infections at VAPHS

"It's hard to gauge the extent of the impact of this new approach to staff engagement because so much of what is happening in the field is informal," explains Kathleen Risa. "But my impression is that there are many, many examples where, when problems arise, the instinct is to get folks together and talk about it and to involve people at all levels of the organization."

Struggles and Triumphs

VAPHS' progress in controlling MRSA has "not been a straight line up," says Chief of Staff Rajiv Jain. "There have been ups and downs. We may take two small steps forward and then comes a long step backward. Units that are MRSA-free today can show infections tomorrow."

He noted: "The move from TPS to PD in 2005 created, at least among some individuals, anger, frustration, and consternation. They felt that their contributions would not be recognized....that they would be sidelined. It was important that TPS be given its due for we would not have been here if it were not for TPS."

Further, with PD making inroads, many VAPHS staff members saw their roles changing, especially as individual and collective responsibility for MRSA prevention increased. For many staff members, especially in infection control, their work burden was now more widely shared. However, for other staff members this was hard; now they no longer could be invisible because their role in infection prevention was defined in addition to all their other responsibilities.

Cheryl Creen, MRSA coordinator at Heinz, added: "Identifying bottlenecks to MRSA prevention is relatively easy for the staff to do. However, how to work around them, or overcome them, in a government agency, is often difficult."

A Ripple Creating a Tidal Wave

The VAPHS' quest to prevent MRSA, supported by measures of its effectiveness, was noticed at the CDC, at the Veterans Health Administration (VHA) in Washington D.C., at the Agency for Health care Research and Quality, and at private granting agencies such as The Robert Wood Johnson Foundation.

On August 17-18, 2006, the VHA administration held a kick-off event in Pittsburgh to launch its national initiative to combat MRSA titled "Getting to Zero," with VAPHS as the lead implementing agency. The effort was led by Rajiv Jain. Carefully-chosen representatives from seventeen VHA hospitals, who had applied to participate in Phase 1 of this national initiative, descended on Pittsburgh for this event.

Since these initial experiments in the VA, the MRSA initiative has grown to include the entire department of 153 hospitals. In January, 2007, Jain was told by the Secretary of Veterans Affairs to roll out, in a matter of months, the MRSA prevention initiative in VA intensive care units across the nation. Since then, all VA hospitals have taken the initiative housewide. Currently, there is a new focus on preventing infections in patients with spinal cord injuries, mental health problems, and those cared for in outpatient facilities.

The core driver of the VAPHS "getting to zero" MRSA Prevention Initiative was "the bundle," comprised of four essential elements: (1) Standard

Precautions: hand hygiene before and after every patient contact; (2) Active Surveillance Cultures: nares swab; at admission, discharge, transfer; (3) Contact Precautions and islation for all MRSA Positive Patients; isolation; hand hygiene, gown, glove, and mask; designated or disinfected equipment; (4) Leadership Support: fostering a culture for transformation from the inside out; setting the direction for the intervention; providing freedom and opportunities for staff to co-create solutions; and eliminating barriers to solving problems encountered by staff. This fourth element of the bundle was informed by VAPHS' experience with Positive Deviance

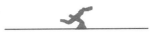

Health care-associated MRSA infections in VA hospital intensive care units have declined by 59 per cent nationally between October 2007 and March 2009.

The strategy for this scaling effort was to tell hospital staff to implement the bundle—to tell them "what to do." But when it came to "how to do it" hospitals would determine that at the local level. Thus some hospitals tapped the PD process while others did not. All hospitals were expected, however, to determine how best to engage front line staff and their expertise, the fourth item in the bundle. Based on experience of what worked in other VA facilities, hospitals were also encouraged to:

- Conduct Discovery and Action Dialogues

- Hold unit briefings once a week (to which everyone is invited)

- Keep the momentum going (schedule regular calls to keep the community feeling supported and connected to each other and to VAPHS).

A tiny ripple of a project, launched serendipitously on the 4 West surgical unit of VAPHS' University Drive Facility in 2002, is generating a large network of activities some years later. And national-level results have been impressive: health care-associated MRSA infections in VA hospital intensive care units have declined by 59 per cent nationally between October 2007 and March 2009.

Further, many VA hospitals have undertaken MRSA prevention initiatives in collaboration with local partners. For example, an initiative at the

Lebanon, PA facility involves women's organizations, local schools and sports teams in partnerships to prevent MRSA.

Overall, the approach has, according to Kathleen Risa, resulted in a culture where "many more people step up and show they are more self-empowered" to contribute not only to the MRSA initiative but to solve other safety problems as well.

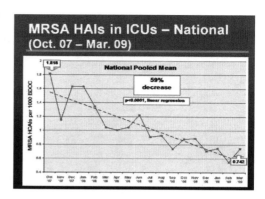

Dramatic declines in MRSA infections in VA hospital intensive care units

Endnotes

1. Edward de Bono, *I Am Right You Are Wrong: From This to the New Renaissance: From Rock Logic to Water Logic,* 1st American edition, (New York: Viking Adult, 1992).

2. Anthony Giddens, *The Constitution of Society: Outline of the Theory of Structuration,* (Berkley: University of California Press, 1986).

Editor Reflections by Curt Lindberg

PD is all about tapping into the expertise within a community and recognizing that the needed knowledge is at our fingertips waiting to be uncovered. The story about the MRSA prevention work at the VA hospital in Pittsburgh is replete with examples. Look how Tanis Smith, a recreational therapist, turned a bingo game into an infection prevention opportunity. Look how a patient, not typically considered sources of guidance in tackling tough problems in hospital operations, helped other veterans understand how infections spread. Darryl observed, "Patients are not the problem. We could be part of the solution." Because the leaders of the MRSA initiative at the hospital recognized that Darryl, and many other people like nurses Jennifer Scott and Cathy Hill, and housekeeper Eddie Yates, had wisdom and experience to offer, he is part of the solution.

In the background material on complexity science covered in Chapter 3, the concept of nonlinearity was introduced. This concept suggests that in complex systems, like hospitals, large changes almost always begin with small actions. In the history of the VA hospital's work we saw how a MRSA initiative begun on one unit, 4 West, eventually led to adoption of the PD process throughout the hospital and inspired many other hospitals across North and South America to join the ranks of PD health care pioneers. Small actions by many people. Stay alert for examples in all the hospital stories and remember that sometimes seemingly insignificant changes end up making a huge difference.

Chapter 5
More We Than Me: Fighting MRSA Inspires a New Way of Collaborating at Albert Einstein Medical Center
by Prucia Buscell

Brief is this existence, like a brief visit in a strange house. The path to be pursued is poorly lit by a flickering consciousness whose center is the limiting and separating 'I'…when a group of individuals becomes a 'we', a harmonious whole, they have reached as high as humans can reach.

— Albert Einstein

Dorothy Borton, a thoughtful woman with a gracious bearing, never liked being considered an enforcer. She is an RN with more than 30 years of clinical experience in infection prevention, and she remembers the way it used to be when she walked onto a hospital unit. "People would make a great show of doing things the correct way, but I got the sense that as soon as I walked away, their actions would change," she said. "If you asked them two years ago who is in charge of infection control, they would say it's the infection control professionals. Now it's recognized that every person in the facility regardless of individual role—the janitor, the finance officer, the direct care giver, patient or visitor—plays a part in preventing infection."

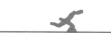

Now it's recognized that every person in the facility regardless of individual role—the janitor, the finance officer, the direct care giver, patient or visitor— plays a part in preventing infection.

That's a big difference. Borton enjoys seeing employees throughout the hospital working together now as a team, and she is especially pleased that infection control professionals are now viewed as a resource, not as police. "It's been fun working with individuals, seeing them grow, and seeing unlikely leaders become advocates and champions," she said. The transition had its discomforts— for her and her colleagues, it meant doing more asking than answering. It also meant giving up some control and becoming comfortable with new and evolving responsibilities.

"The whole landscape of infection control has changed in the last two or three years," Borton observed. "We're much more visible now. The appearance of H1N1 showed that—all the messages were about hand hygiene and social distancing. There have been changes in the way we deal with employee illness. In the past you were a hero if you dragged your sick body in to work. Now we say stay home—we don't want you here with your infections. That kind of summarizes how things have changed."

Innovations in a Changed Landscape

Borton's increasingly collaborative relationship with physicians, nurses and ancillary staff is part of a journey that Albert Einstein Healthcare Network began in 2006. Albert Einstein, a nonprofit organization with 6,000 employees and several major facilities and outpatient centers in the Philadelphia area, embarked on a new infection fighting strategy that has changed relationships and workplace habits among countless health professionals and other employees. The incidence of health care-associated Methicillin resistant *Staphylococcus aureus* (MRSA) and other infections has been reduced, and interestingly, as the rates drop, the percentage of staph infections caused by the drug resistant bacteria has also declined.

Further, Einstein, in cooperation with other hospitals and the federal Centers for Disease Control and Prevention (CDC) helped pioneer important new tools that health care organizations nationally can use to measure the effectiveness of their MRSA prevention efforts. In May 2006 the CDC ran training sessions in Atlanta to teach participants how to use a new MRSA surveillance system. It was the first of its kind in the country, and it came about through an unusual collaboration. Trish Perl, MD, professor of medicine, pathology and epidemiology at The Johns Hopkins Hospital, worked with in-

It's been fun working with individuals, seeing them grow, and seeing unlikely leaders become advocates and champions.

fection control professionals at six U.S. Beta Site hospitals in collaboration with John Jernigan, MD, the CDC's then acting deputy chief of prevention and response, and his CDC colleagues. The new surveillance system let the six hospitals collect and submit uniform data on MRSA infections. It is now part of the CDC's National Healthcare Safety Network (NHSN) and available to any hospital in the U.S. that wants to use it.

The six hospitals, plus two from Colombia, were partners in testing a behavioral change process used to fight infection. That effort was set in motion in February 2006, when Jeffrey Cohn, MD, chief quality officer at Einstein, and Borton learned about The Robert Wood Johnson Foundation grant to support a pioneering effort by Plexus Institute and the Positive Deviance Initiative to use Positive Deviance (PD) to fight MRSA. The idea is that PD, which does not rely on new drugs or technology, encourages the kinds of cultural changes that help people consistently adhere to practices known to fight infections. Presenters at a "kick-off" meeting hosted by the Hospital Council of Western Pennsylvania included Curt Lindberg and the late Jerry Sternin, the leading international authority on PD and the director of the Positive Deviance Initiative, who outlined the opportunities for using PD in health care; John A. Jernigan, MD, a medical epidemiologist with CDC who described dangers of MRSA, and representatives from Veterans Administration Pittsburgh Healthcare System (VAPHS), who told how they had piloted the use of PD in MRSA prevention. Cohn and Borton were there and were captivated. Borton, who also serves on the Healthcare Associated Infections Advisory Panel of the Pennsylvania Patient Safety Authority, remembers Cohn was on his cell phone planning the start of Einstein's program before their homeward flight out of Pittsburgh.

"We knew that the percentage of MRSA isolates cultured in our microbiology lab was steadily increasing, we noticed that isolation lists kept getting longer, and that health care-acquired MRSA infections occurred more frequently," Borton recalled. "And the timing was right. We had just started a transformational process, and this dovetailed wonderfully into that, with a different approach."

"We had talked about connecting more with what is happening on the front lines, and getting a much greater sense of engagement and ownership among those who are on the front lines," Cohn said. "And PD as a tool is all about the front lines. I was convinced if we could learn to do this well, it would be in complete alignment with our transformational work."

Einstein invited several hundred executives, managers and department heads as well as doctors, and nurses and support staff to a "kick-off" session in the spring of 2006. Cohn shared his own wrenching MRSA story. Some years earlier, when he was a practicing oncologist, he treated a college professor in his 50s who had been diagnosed with a serious but treatable cancer. The prognosis was years of remission. Instead, the man died of lung failure resulting from a blood stream MRSA infection that he almost certainly got through an IV line put in place for chemotherapy. "It was devastating for the family and as the doc who had embarked him on this treatment, I felt horrible," Cohn said. An Einstein board member told of his experience with a *staph aureus* infection. Jerry Zuckerman, MD, Einstein's medical director of infection prevention and control, outlined what MRSA bacteria is and does. David Hares, MD, an internal medicine physician who recently earned an MBA at the University of Michigan, had served an internship with a biotech company trying to develop a MRSA treatment. He had become Einstein's quality manager just days earlier, but he quickly joined the session, recounting the numbers of people MRSA sickened and killed. Jerry Sternin and his colleague and wife Monique Sternin talked about Positive Deviance and how it had worked in health care. As the session ended, Cohn invited anyone interested in volunteering to help in the new fight against MRSA to come to a session at 9 AM the next day.

"We were very nervous," Cohn recalled. "Would anyone show up?" A circle of a dozen chairs initially went unoccupied as a few people straggled into the room a little after 9 AM. "Einstein time," scoffed several doctors who noted that meetings often start late. Eventually, some 50 doctors, nurses, aides, administrators, housekeepers, and clergy were among those who brought more chairs to join the circle. The conversations started that day would grow into a concerted effort involving hundreds of people. Pilot projects began in four units and people who work with patients in numerous capacities throughout the hospital began to re-examine their own roles and the way they worked with others to prevent infections.

"We were very nervous," Cohn recalled. "Would anyone show up?" Eventually, some 50 doctors, nurses, aides, administrators, housekeepers, and clergy were among those who brought more chairs to join the circle.

"I think we were able to see some complexity principles at work in that first hour or two," Cohn said in retrospect. "There was self-organization, and people without a clear agenda saying how do we proceed, how do we make sense of this next task. Within 30 to 40 minutes, people had self-organized into subgroups." Some would be short-lived, such as a group who worked on early logistics, and other groups would continue working on such issues as measurement, communication and support for the pilot units.

Early Skeptics

Despite dedication and enthusiasm, the initiative did not come together with magical ease or speed. Many were skeptical then, and Cohn concedes some still are.

Zuckerman became the physician champion for SMASH. That's an acronym for Stop MRSA Acquisition and Spread in our Hospitals, the name staff members voted to call the PD MRSA initiative. Hares, a PD enthusiast, was project manager for SMASH. Zuckerman was an early skeptic. "I asked where is the evidence, where is the science?" he remembered. "The science and the guidelines tell us what we should all be doing for infection prevention and control. However, despite universal knowledge of best practices, health care workers routinely fail to follow them. PD is a very different process. It strives to invoke behavioral and cultural changes. It focuses on the 'how' to implement best infection prevention practices, an area that infection control professionals have struggled with for a long time."

Despite his qualms, Zuckerman was swayed by the preliminary reduction in infection rates. He also thinks the PD approach has contributed to increased cooperation, teamwork and involvement of front line staff. In the summer of 2007 he observed, "We've made more progress on this in the last six months than we have in the last 14 years."

Elaine Flynn, RN, the infection control professional for Moss Rehab, which includes Einstein's 30-bed brain injury unit at Elkins Park, was interested early because 29 per cent of the patients arriving in her unit already had MRSA infections or colonizations, and there had been a recent outbreak. Further, because the goal is to return patients to their communities, social and group activities are encouraged, and they spend little time in their rooms. Isolation is unworkable. "These patients are medically very complex, and most have had surgical interventions and lengthy stays in acute care before they get to us," she explained. But she too was an early skeptic. She expected lectures at that May morning meeting, but instead Cohn and Hares asked questions. "I was doubtful. I thought they were trying to get information from us, and I suspected their motives," she said later. But then she realized that people who get questions can give answers. She and a dozen colleagues agreed the brain injury unit should start a pilot program.

When Should We Start? How About Now?

The other pilot units were the surgical intensive care unit (SICU), Tower 8, a 20-bed oncology and transplant unit, and Levy 4W, a "step-down" unit, where patients are seriously ill and suffer from many types of organ failure. Melissa Morris, RN, the Levy 4W nurse manager, says many patients were arriving with *Clostridium difficile*-associated diarrhea, caused by a virulent infection known as C-diff, and Vancomycin-resistant *enterococci*, or VRE, as well as MRSA. "We weren't screening (on admission), but we would discover it later. We knew if we could control it on entry we could do better," Morris said. Morris's then 20-year-old son had suffered from a MRSA infection that required three rounds of incision and drainage procedures and antibiotics, and a nurse on the unit had also endured incision and drainage procedures to treat a MRSA infection. "We had actually seen the effects, so we felt passionately about this," she said.

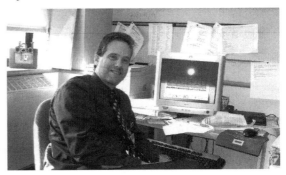

Jerry Zuckerman, MD, an early skeptic, sees more teamwork and fewer infections.

The efforts unfolded differently in each unit. In the brain injury unit, there was an emphasis on educating patients, families and visitors about MRSA facts and infection prevention. Some patients hadn't been told or didn't remember they had MRSA. Morris says active surveillance showed nearly 20 per cent of Levy 4W patients were colonized with MRSA, but not infected, when they arrived. "We wouldn't have known about that, and those patients would have been in with other patients instead of in isolation," she said. While the incidence of all other infections has not been formally analyzed, Morris

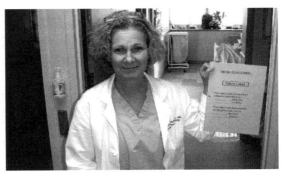

Melissa Morris, RN, shows a new pink form used to let staff know the status of patient screenings for MRSA. A medical clerk came up with the idea.

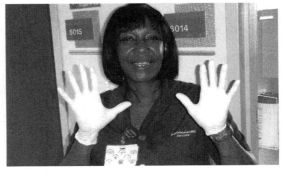

Wanda Davis, Housekeeper on Tower 8, a true positive deviant

observed, "If you're doing prevention you are protecting patients against all of them."

A fifth unit, Levy 7, a 46-bed medical surgical unit, joined SMASH in August. Gene Spross, RN, the nurse manager, had been going to SMASH meetings early on. She intuitively liked PD, but wondered if it could work in her unit, with its 80 employees in two physically separated sections. Still, she kept learning. "My staff knew something exciting was going on, and they wanted to be part of it," she said. "They were honest when they met with Dr. Hares—they said we know we don't always do everything we should. Dr. Hares asked, when do you think you could start this process? Four or five answered 'how about right now'?" SMASH participants go out of their way to help each other. Spross is being mentored in her efforts by Dallas Douglass, RN, nurse manager of Tower 8, who in turn was mentored by Melissa Morris.

And Morris believes helping is part of the process: "When one unit is successful it motivates other units. So they step up and do it, and those who have already worked on it will support them."

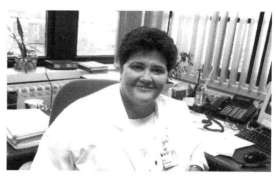

Gene Spross, RN, found the staff enthusiastic about starting PD on her large unit.

On all SMASH units, every patient is screened for MRSA, first upon admission, and then upon transfer to another unit, discharge from the hospital, or death. The MRSA test is conducted by a nasal swab, which is processed in the hospital laboratory. Patients who test positive for MRSA are put in isolation, and staff who enter their

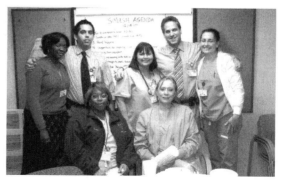

DAD meeting in SICU

rooms are to wear gowns and gloves. Vigilant hand hygiene means all staff members must wash their hands or use hand sanitizer before and after every contact with every patient, regardless of MRSA status. Every patient room has hand hygiene pumps, which also appear in hallways. Sanitizing gel for hands is ubiquitous.

Regular Meetings and Butterflies

Discovery and Action Dialogues, or DADs, as they came to be called, were scheduled as needed on the units. Some dialogues were spontaneous one-on-one exchanges. Some were short bursts of engagement among staff members and mentors. The idea was to talk about an issue, discover whether anyone has already come up with uncommon strategies to address it, and if not, then create an action plan that is as concrete as possible. Volunteers are sought to see that specific steps are carried out. No ideas are ridiculed or dismissed. Ideas are "butterflies" to be examined with care and treated gently. In one DAD with respiratory therapists, participants worried that pens they carried in and out of the rooms might be vectors for transmissions, so pens were to be purchased to keep in isolation rooms. Morris reported that during a DAD with her staff on Levy 4W, a medical clerk came up with the idea of having a pink sheet on all patient bedside charts that showed MRSA status and swab-in, swab-out data. The admission "swab-ins" were accomplished efficiently, but "swab-outs" proved more difficult to do routinely because the transfers and discharges are often rushed and unpredictably timed. Staff experimented with ways to make the swab-outs more consistent.

DADs were to become central to PD work in other hospitals. They allowed for community discussions and elicited a host of suggested solutions. In addition, brief facilitated conversations alleviated the need for big meetings that were hard to schedule in a hectic environment where shift work covers 24 hours. Facilitators at DADs asked these questions:

- How do you know or recognize when MRSA is present?

- How do YOU protect yourself, patients and others from MRSA transmissions?

- What prevents you from taking these actions all the time?

- Is there any group or anyone you know who is able to overcome the barriers frequently and effortlessly? How?

- Do you have any ideas?

- What initial steps need to be pursued to make it happen? Any volunteers?

- Who else needs to be involved?

Jeff Cohn, Jerry Zuckerman, Dorothy Borton or David Hares generally attend regular Friday meetings where staff from pilot units discusses their progress with prevention, barriers to prevention, and possible solutions. The sessions are open, and members of several units and support services are invited or attend on their own. After months of practice, discussions at the Friday meetings flowed easily, with partners in conversation augmenting each other's observations and proposals. Coaches, including Jon

For Ideas and Butterflies: Gentle Hands

From the burweed
such a butterfly
was born!
—Issa[1]

Jerry and Monique Sternin, pioneers of Positive Deviance, liked to emphasize that ideas are like butterflies. They need to be caught gently, and allowed to live and breathe, never crushed or stifled. Sometimes, the strength and beauty of an idea isn't obvious when it is born. Like the chrysalis, it has to grow its bright colored wings to take flight. Sometimes it takes three generations of butterflies to complete the Monarchs' arduous annual migration. And sometimes it takes many iterations for an emerging idea to be honed for a specific purpose.

Each year swarms of Monarch butterflies travel thousands of miles in perilous journeys from Canada and North America to southern California and the mountains of Mexico. It's an astonishing feat for creatures that weigh less than an ounce and have very tiny primitive brains. Yet they are among the few living creatures able to orient themselves by latitude and longitude—something human sailors didn't manage until the seventeenth century with the help of clocks, sextants and the compass. Entomologists aren't sure how butterflies do it. Equally amazing is that their marathon migration is multi-generational. Many don't live long enough to complete the whole trip. But the urgency of their purpose outlasts individual lifespans. Butterflies that reach the Mexican mountains in the fall are likely to be second and third generation descendants of the Monarchs that began their flights the

Lloyd, MD, the late Jerry Sternin, consultant Sharon Benjamin from Plexus Institute and Plexus Chair Henri Lipmanowicz, often participated in regular conference calls about PD and infection issues.

The Friday meetings were continuing in early 2010, Zuckerman said, and the use of PD and DADs have permeated other initiatives. "Our urinary tract infection group finds out from front line people what some of the problems are, and they are being very inclusive, working with a bottom up approach, and incorporating those ideas into clinical areas and projects."

Nothing About Me Without Me

"The complexity of taking care of patients, of hundreds of interactions every day, in a complex environment, that's where PD comes into play,"

preceding spring. Donald McNeil, in his *New York Times* story "Fly Away Home," describes the extraordinary durability of these delicate creatures as they evade predators and survive battering winds and rain. He writes that whether Monarchs lift off from Maine or Montana, success in reaching the mountains of Mexico means "threading a geographic needle" by passing through a 50-mile gap of river valleys in Texas.[2] An idea, too, can survive and travel in surprising ways to reach resolution of a workplace problem.

In a hospital where infection fighters were trying to instill the culture of consistent gown and glove use during every contact with patients who had MRSA, it appeared that adherence among clinical staff was only about 30 per cent. They discussed how that could be improved. One nurse observed, "If I can count my son's underwear to make sure he is changing,

we can do this." Measurement was key, they decided, so they collected data on gown usage and displayed it publicly on graphs where all clinical staff could see it. Eventually, the data they gathered would be able to show a connection between proper use of personal protective gear and declining infections. The child's underwear count was the chrysalis. Nurtured and discussed among a group of health care professionals, the idea became a butterfly, a surprisingly flexible and natural solution to a workplace challenge.

Notes

1. R. H. Blyth, *Haiku, Volume 1, Eastern Culture*, (Hokuseido: Japan, 1949), 253.

2. D. McNeil, "Fly Away Home," *The New York Times*, October 3, 2006. http://www.nytimes.com/2006/10/03/science/03butter.html?_r=3&ref=science&oref=slogin (accessed 5-20-10).

said Zuckerman. "With the traditional approach, leadership gets an idea of what's wrong and imposes a solution. The natural reaction is 'that won't work for us.' PD is about people in the community identifying the problems you can't see from the outside, and coming up with novel ideas that work for them, right there. It's about community ownership. Because solutions are community driven, they are likely to be accepted. People don't throw away their own babies.

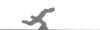

"*Housekeeping and transport have folks who care passionately about the role they play in preventing infection. The people in the store room where supplies are kept have played important roles.*"

"If the discussion involves another person or another group, they have to be brought in," Zuckerman continued. "That's how you expand the community. If you don't know how a room is cleaned, you bring in housekeeping." Employees from several departments, including food services, radiology, patient transport and therapy became vigilant infection fighters and found multiple ways to remove barriers to their own consistent vigilance. In fact, Cohn notes that some of the people Jerry Sternin calls "unusual suspects", the people who have not traditionally been invited to work on infection control, are among Einstein's "heroes." "Environmental Services (housekeeping) and transport have folks who care passionately and have tremendous pride in the role they can play in preventing infection," Cohn says. "The people in the store room where supplies are kept have played important roles."

Supplies were a major issue when SMASH began. There weren't enough gowns, or gloves, or they were the wrong sizes, or nurses and doctors thought they were too hot or poorly designed. After considerable research on different designs, 400 staff members voted that the original gowns were the best. But then there was the matter of availability. "Lack of equipment was identified as a barrier to infection control," said Dallas Douglass, of Tower 8. "Sometimes you'd see gowns hanging on the back of doors because people intended to re-use them. That's no good." Store rooms weren't always fully stocked, and closed cabinets prolonged searches. Some units tried keeping supplies in boxes on tables in the hallways. But that created clutter. Douglass said a staff member suggested an enormously helpful solution: Plexiglas supply boxes now adorn the walls outside every patient room in all SMASH units. The supplies, swabs for nasal MRSA tests, gowns, and gloves in boxes color coded for size, are handy and visible. "My staff is doing a great job," Douglass said. "Nurses and aides are very acutely aware of supplies, and they keep those boxes filled. No one waits for someone else to do it." Borton says those boxes became coveted items, and now they are used throughout the hospital. And nurses and aides still keep them stocked, without anyone needing to be assigned.

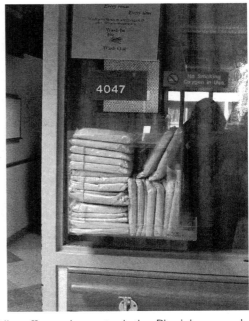

All staff members stock the Plexiglass supply cabinets outside each room, where gowns, gloves and nasal swabs are handy and visible.

"You can see the teamwork growing," Douglass reflected. "People from other units ask the staff questions about how we are doing. And there is less friction. No one gets ruffled about a reminder on hand hygiene or gowning and gloving." She calls herself a "true believer" in PD, which she says fits well with the shared governance that has been in place for 10 years among Einstein nurses.

The use of patient transport "improvs" illustrates how teamwork evolved along with refinements in PD processes. When SMASH began, there had been complaints about transporters from escort service walking around the hospital in contaminated gowns, said Maureen Jordan, administrative director of respiratory care. So they took them off. But who should wear them, and when? A therapist had raised questions. The CDC had no specific policy on wearing protective gear during in-house transports. The first improv, involved a nurse, an escort, an oxygen tank and ventilator, and Jerry Zuckerman on a stretcher playing a creatively noncompliant critically-ill patient. Jordan took notes, and was amazed to discover the number of previously unrecognized opportunities for microbial transmission.

Under a new policy that resulted, a nurse who prepares the patient for transport removes the gown worn inside the patient room. The respiratory therapist, who may have to adjust a patient's breathing tube, always wears gown and gloves. The patient is draped with a clean sheet so that any equipment or oxygen cylinders placed on the stretcher won't touch contaminated bedding. The section of the bed or stretcher that will be touched for the transport is wiped with a disinfectant wipe prior to exiting the room. The escort, who does not wear protective gear, won't touch the patient, but will push the stretcher (touching the disinfected area), push buttons to open doors and elevators, and touch anything else that needs to be moved. At the end of the transport, the receiving team gets information about the infection status of the patient and is prepared to gown and glove in the patient's room. The details were worked out by front line staff with guidance from Dorothy Borton. Jordan said the exercise had reduced awareness of hierarchies, improved relationships among people who hadn't previously collaborated, and made everyone more observant of their own roles.

The PD approach is to acknowledge the expertise of those who do the work. It is also flexible enough to address new issues and revisit old ones. As it turned out, there were still more questions about the best methods for in-house transports.

Denise Kirby is a registered respiratory therapist who accepted Maureen Jordan's designation as the department's SMASH representative. When Hares addressed the department about MRSA, Kirby asked: "We gown and glove when we go into the patient's room. When we take the ventilator patient to a study, we take the stuff off. Why? We're still interacting with the patient?"

Acting Out, With Post-Its

Hares wasn't sure and invited Kirby to look into it. She observed transports and investigated how other hospitals did it. She searched the internet, and called the Infectious Disease Department at Johns Hopkins. "I saw they used a 'clean' person when transporting," she said. "I got information from them, then started getting to work." Zuckerman calls Kirby a true positive deviant and SMASH champion.

Kirby and colleagues focused on transporting critically-ill patients, who needed ventilators and other equipment with them and were always accompanied by a nurse. They started by watching, asking questions and trying to find out anything they might be inadvertently doing wrong. They began improvs, with different employees playing the role of

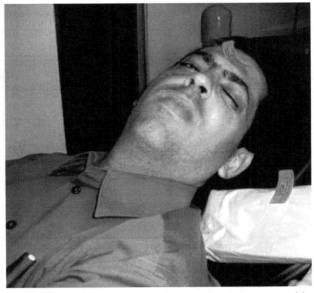

David Hares, MD, plays a patient being transported in the hospital. Post-It Notes pasted on his face and body show where a patient might have had inadvertent contact with germs.

nurse, respiratory therapist, transport workers and patient. They did more than a dozen inprovs, and each time they came up with a suggested change, they'd act it out in another improv to see what really worked, and what might go wrong. Nursing, infection control, physical therapy, operating room, and radiology staffs were involved. "Radiology had a big impact on our eventual policy," Kirby said. "Patents would get to radiology, and they wouldn't know what kind of isolation they were on. SMASH is for MRSA, but there are other isolations that have other procedures. So we had to correct that. When a patient is in isolation, the chart goes into a black bag, and a sleeve on the chart identifies the type of isolation the patient is on and what precautions to take."

"On one transport there were more than 20 opportunities for cross-contamination," she recalled. "I never thought there could be that many. Everything you did was a potential source—holding the chart, opening a door, touching the side of the bed. When Dr. Hares played the role of the noncompliant patient, we put Post-Its on him every time some member of the team touched him or an area where there was a potential for infection transmission. At the end of the exercise there were Post-Its all over him."

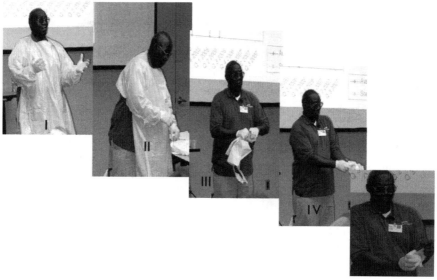

Jasper Palmer demonstrating the "Palmer Method" for removing and compressing a used hospital gown.

Kirby explains: "You're ventilating the patient, and he's moving all around, and you're saying *stay still*, and you touch the nurse with the IV, then you touch the elevator button. You touch the patient's forehead without a gloved hand. Interestingly, we thought you weren't allowed to wear gowns and gloves in the hallways, and we found that was a misinterpretation of the regulations. The idea is that can't go into a patient's room with gowns and gloves, and then come out to the nurses station and talk, but you can keep them on if you are continuously caring for the patient. So it was the hospital learning too."

Their innovations for learning included a brief film showing the "wrong" and "right" way to do a transport, to the tune of Pink Floyd's "We Don't Need No Education." A safe and successful transport has instrumental accompaniment. It took more than a year to write a new policy that spelled out every step in detail. Their directions include an innovation created by another positive deviant colleague. Transport worker Jasper Palmer devised a way to slip out of a hospital gown, role it tightly and stuff it into a glove, thereby reducing risk of infection from contact with contaminated gear as well as shrinking the volume of trash.

A Rocky Start and "Huge" Achievement

Cohn thinks the SMASH program in SICU may have had an especially rough start because it was started by leaders without strong community ownership. A cultural collision also may have impeded progress. "The SICU nurses are very skilled and very tough," observed Hares, who helped facilitate SICU meetings. "They are not touchy-feely. When we went to SICU and asked what do you feel, what do you think, that was a mismatch. Their culture is you tell us a better way and we will carry it out."

Karen Niewood, RN, the clinical manager for SICU, says members of the unit initially suspected SMASH was another "initiative of the week" that would soon fade. Further, they doubted that MRSA could be eradicated. "Our patients are critically ill. They need very intensive, often very immediate, interventions to save their lives. Swabbing for MRSA just didn't seem like the highest priority. When Dr. Hares and Dr. Zuckerman first approached us we were skeptical." she said. She paused, and

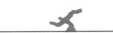

"Our patients are critically ill. Swabbing for MRSA just didn't seem like the highest priority. But if you save someone from a motor vehicle accident, and they die two months later from an infection, you ask yourself what else could have been done."

then added, "But if you save someone from a motor vehicle accident, and they die two months later from an infection, you ask yourself what else could have been done?" Niewood began researching the literature on MRSA, and attending meetings to learn what other units were doing. She shared her knowledge and the articles with colleagues. As a result of a SICU SMASH meeting, a unit bulletin board proclaims "SMASH in Action: 95% swab in, 95% swab out." The absence of central-line associated bloodstream infections is another initiative, Niewood notes, but many principles are the same as SMASH—hand hygiene and use of protective gear. Hares says Niewood was instrumental in bringing about change in SICU, because of her competence, generosity with time and effort, and her ability to encourage people to find a few minutes for conversation.

Nancy Pokorny, RN, a nursing career specialist, also met with SICU and agrees the unit was a "tough nut to crack" for SMASH. The fast-paced stressful ICU has its own culture. Jon Lloyd, a surgeon, and others had listened to a discussion of whether efforts should be continued to involve SICU staff in SMASH. Pokorny suggested they might be more accepting of someone with a surgical trauma background. She also urged Hares to tell the staff that he had experience in critical care. "I thought they needed a surgeon for credibility," she said. When Lloyd got Jerry Zuckerman's message proclaiming there had been no clinical MRSA infection for 88 days and no transmissions for 44 days, he re-

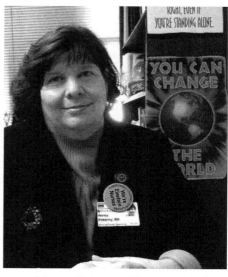

Nancy Pokorny, RN, says the fast-paced, stressful ICU was a "tough nut to crack."

sponded, "Congratulations to the SICU Marines. Semper Fi."

When the initiative started, Pokorny says, the staff thought nurses were being targeted to the exclusion of others who have contact with patients. She remembers one meeting with six or eight nurses that became especially tense when a nurse from a different critical care unit stood in the doorway, declining an invitation to enter the meeting room, and provocatively demanded to know why Zuckerman was the only physician present. The nurse, whose clinical manager had sent him to the meeting, may have assumed that a colleague was being unfairly blamed for a MRSA transmission. A MRSA transmission was being discussed, Pokorny recalled, but the focus was on how it might have happened, not who was at fault. The nurse said nurses should receive bonuses for preventing infections, and Zuckerman mildly suggested he come up with a business model.

Pokorny was disturbed afterwards. She considered the bonus notion unethical, even though she suspected the exchange was at least an opening to get more people involved. At the same time, she sensed there remained distrust for the PD process and the sharing of thoughts, feelings, and actual practices in the group process. "*Nothing about me without me* leaves only me or us to talk about," she elaborated. "That can be difficult to do initially in these groups, even though they work together." She recalled Zuckerman stressing the importance of continued meetings and dialogue. Zuckerman now says the "us against them" attitude between doctors and nurses is gone, and his sentiment is confirmed by several other staff members. Zuckerman observed that people in the hospital community have become far more comfortable reminding each other about hand hygiene.

Very gradually, through dialogue, meetings and action, the SICU achieved tremendous change. According to David Hares the staff interacted more and created their own shared agenda. Zuckerman said no HA-MRSA infections for three months is "huge" for a surgical ICU, and he added he's been told more people there are "looking out for each other, and that assumes more people are doing the right things." Pokorny thinks a turning point came when Zuckerman told the SICU staff, "We're here to help, facilitate and guide, but this is your community. You guys have to decide whether you want to do this." In discussion that followed, SICU responded as a community, and staff members began facilitating their own meetings.

Jeff Cohn thinks two crises helped bring the staff together. On October 31, 2007, a Philadelphia police officer was shot in the head during a robbery at a nearby Dunkin' Donuts and brought to Einstein for emergency surgery to remove a bullet from his brain. The officer never regained consciousness, and died some 36 hours later. "It was a very emotionally intense thing for the staff, and those grieving for the officer. The staff did a fantastic job, and they were lauded by the media and the officer's family," Cohn said, so despite their sadness, they could take pride in their work. Around the same time, Cohn said, a much-loved physician was a SICU patient for two or three weeks, with several potential portals where infection could have entered his body. "They took perfect care of him," Cohn commented. "I think both of these events opened their eyes to the work they have always been delivering but in less publicly recognized ways."

The Numbers Are Heartfelt

Lloyd always says PD is "bathed in data." And as Zuckerman put it, ongoing measurements reinforce change. Staff members at Einstein take the numbers very personally.

Elaine Flynn kept a grid over a 63-week period of transmission and infection rates in the brain injury unit. In December 2007, when the unit had gone nine weeks without a new MRSA infection, the staff rejoiced. "Then there was a transmission, and everyone was really down," she remembered. "We all felt bad. When that happens, we go over it to see what we could have done to prevent it." Nurses on other units confirm good numbers feel good and a transmission brings disappointment and self examination. "We're here to help people, not infect them," asserted Dallas Douglass. "When they see a downward trend in infections and transmissions, the staff can see the whole continuum of their work and what it means to people."

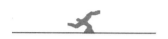

"We're here to help people, not to infect them."

The SMASH units keep records of MRSA infections, colonizations, and transmissions. Hand hygiene adherence rates, often based on observance by an unidentified outsider, are also recorded. Karen Niewood of SICU and other nurses think there is value in having staff members record the data by hand. It attaches the numbers to individuals. Lloyd notes ownership of the data is vital. "This is not a report card," he says. "When staff create the solutions they realize that performance data reflect changes they are making and the solutions they are implementing, and that they own the data, And the data answer what all health care workers die to know: 'how are we doing'?"

Zuckerman cautions that it is almost impossible to pinpoint where a specific transmission occurs. But he lauds the sense of individual responsibility that encourages people to strive to do what's right. Ultimately, he says, that's what makes for the best infection control.

"I think that before no one believed they were spreading infection," Melissa Morris observed. "But when you do the hand hygiene, and the gowns and the gloves, and do the data, the results are really noticeable."

Cohn notes that literature and Einstein's own analysis shows patients who acquired MRSA are more expensive to treat than patients with similar conditions who do not have MRSA infections. But he says clinical outcomes, not cost, are the rationale for Einstein's program. The CDC estimates the overall annual direct medical cost of health care-associated infections to U.S. hospitals ranges from $35.7 billion to $45 billion.

Can SMASH Achievements Be Sustained?

When a prominent infectious disease professor asked this question at a Phildelphia-wide infection prevention symposium in November 2007, several Einstein front line employees were indignant. Of course infection control vigilance will last, several insisted, because they will make it last. It is their process.

The plans for a network-wide SMASH program offer some insights on maintaining an effort. The decision had many roots. Doctors making rounds were noticing SMASH units were better than others at having personal protective gear available, and staff more consistently followed hand hygiene and isolation precautions. Gene Spross and Dallas Douglass and several other nurses were beginning to think SMASH should be universal. Hares and Carlos Urrea, MD, another quality management physician, and Dorothy Borton, the infection control nurse, were starting conversations with additional units. Cohn says a joint decision was reached in the spring of 2007 to expand the initiative. "We all looked at what we were doing, and uncovering, and the value of making all these previously invisible MRSA patients visible, and knowing our patient population, and we knew it was the right thing to do," Cohn said. "Then the state mandated MSRA testing for high risk patients. We have a lot of people from long-term care, or chronic renal failure, who would be viewed as high risk. It just made sense." As Hares put it, "It was a desire, not a decision. It was a request from people who were a part of SMASH, who said we have something good and we have to share it. It was discussed, and expressed, and shared with others, and that's how the desire became a decision."

There was some initial resistance, he said, "But the beauty of PD is the concept of *unusual suspects*. If the usual suspects are too busy, or unconcerned, move to the next person. And eventually the usual suspects will comply because someone asks them to. People resist, then they get sucked into a big movement. Nothing was ever imposed. People find their own way."

As of January 2010, he said, 93 per cent of all patients in the hospital have known MRSA status after they are admitted.

The majority of Einstein's patients are admitted through the Emergency Department. In DADs held with the department leadership, staff came up with procedures, and now every patient is tested. Cohn had grappled with the question of how to use PD while mandating compliance, and says he has not come up with a perfect answer. He says, for instance, that it made sense for wall cabinets that make supplies visible to be used house-wide, and it wasn't necessary to let each unit discover they needed them.

"We've taken the spread of SMASH to all of our stakeholders to say this is what needs to happen: we will do surveillance cultures on all our admissions not known to be already colonized," he explained. "We say we want to help you understand how to dialogue with your staff, and know how it will impact on them, so you can give them a choice of how it is getting started in their micro system. But the decision to do it is not an option."

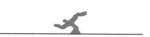

People resist, then they get sucked into a big movement. Nothing was ever imposed. People find their own way.

Borton thinks most staff members will gladly sustain the effort because the news stories, public attention, and in-house efforts have raised awareness and made the importance very clear. "Besides," she says, "It's the 'in' thing to do."

Several Einstein staff members think changed relationships and a sense of ownership will support continuation of newly developed infection control practices and behavior. Maureen Jordan offers a similar observation, and cites her own personal changes. Hares observes that because of continual work-related conversations, people from different units and occupations communicate more freely: "More people know each other on a first-name basis," he commented.

Maureen Jordan, a self-described Type A personality, tells how her attitudes and relationships have changed. "I was used to identifying a problem and getting the correction implemented, 1, 2, 3," she said. " Here's my time line, let's get this done. But then, three months later, the same problem would be happening and people would be doing things the old way. Now it's not just me preaching. It's people feeling they have created something that they own."

Even language has changed. Several Einstein employees have noticed that people at all levels of the organization address each other more respectfully, and that speech is more inclusive. Most respond politely to reminders about MRSA prevention practices, no matter the source. Borton notes nurses offer reminders graciously, and doctors tend to be pleasantly unflummoxed. Zuckerman summarizes the change with the observation, "there's more 'we' than 'me'."

Swab-in and swab-out aren't in standard dictionaries yet, and stories have a whole new meaning. "If you are in a meeting and you say you have a story to share, you are no longer the crazy guy," Hares said. "They are a part of what we do today. Even a vice president told a story about something that she experienced, and how she solved it, and it was a springboard for discussion." Another newly frequent phrase is "I don't know, let's ask," Hares added. And butterflies? A new metaphor, it doesn't signify queasy stomachs or flighty socializing, but rather inspiration, ideas and practical solutions. "When we talk about butterflies we mean ideas that are floating over the middle of the table," explained an Einstein nurse at a meeting of health care professionals. "When there is a butterfly, someone has to catch it, not strangle it, or squash it, but catch it and work on it." Several staffers

Even language has changed. Several employees have noticed that people at all levels of the organization address each other more respectfully, and that speech is more inclusive. "There's more 'we' than 'me'."

have favorite butterfly stories. Hares recalls one that brought about some specific new practices. Carlos Urrea was meeting with a new unit not yet formally in SMASH. He asked staff members to write down what they were doing to prevent infection. "One nurse said she wipes her shoes with Sani-wipes when she leaves the hospital," Hares recalled. "That was to protect her family, but Carlos asked what does it mean here? The nurse manager used that story and it led to wiping down many more pieces of equipment on the unit with disinfectant wipes. That was a butterfly."

PD processes are being used to address other issues. Borton said a group working to reduce blood stream infections used PD to examine processes, products and practices involved in infection prevention. A group working to prevent C-diff used PD, and another group working to prevent urinary tract infections used the PD process to create a multi-disciplinary team, identify who needs to be in the discussion, what needs to be done and what are the obstacles. The team is producing a check list for indications of who actually needs a urinary catheter, and every step needed to prevent patient infections, Hares said, and reports from summer of 2009 showed urinary tract infections and central line infections are down.

Hand hygiene is not a standard reportable item, Borton said, so meaningful statistics are hard to come by. However, she expects that it will eventually be incorporated into many more areas and become part of written "bundles" subject to observation and documentation. "One of the things we have evolving here is more people who are willing to be role models, who are willing to say to a colleague, 'you forgot something'," Borton said. "We have a couple of physician leaders who say to their staffs, 'if I don't do hand hygiene, it's your responsibility to remind me.' That's part of the culture change we've had here, that rank doesn't matter when it's the right thing to do."

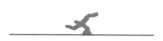

Stories have a whole new meaning. "If you are in a meeting and you say you have a story to share, you are no longer the crazy guy," Hares said. "They are a part of what we do today."

Leadership has changed too, she notes, and more attention is paid to attitudes on the front lines. Hospital executives recently approved a switch from hand gel to foam in dispensers throughout the building, despite additional expense, even though the cleaning power of both products is the same. But people like the foam better, Borton said, because it dries faster and doesn't feel as sticky. "The feeling was if it is more acceptable to staff, they will use it more frequently and we will have improved hand hygiene," she said. In the past, expense alone would have been an obstacle to change.

David Hares said in addition to changed habits and practices, the long-term impact of the PD MRSA work includes obtaining an external grant of $24,000 from Cardinal Healthcare. This grant will allow Kirby and colleagues to work on disseminating the new policies for in-house transport of critically ill isolation patients. The grant provides for a person to facilitate sessions day and night for 800 employees—nurses, aides, transport, radiology, therapists, all the support and ancillary people. Hares recently left his position as SMASH project manager. He completed a residency in internal medicine in Argentina and has started residency here, but his influence remains strong. The team has evaluated its role and developed the following purpose statement: "Our purpose as the SMASH team is to *facilitate the development* of processes and systems for sustainable behavior to eliminate hospital-acquired infections. We do this *using a positive deviance methodology*, incorporating patient and staff perspectives, and *including as many people as we can in the process*." Where this expanded focus will lead the team is to be determined; ongoing evidence of complexity at work.

Editor Reflections by Curt Lindberg

The Einstein story begins with reflections from Dorothy Borton about how challenging it was for her, an infection control specialist, to let go of control and share infection-prevention responsibilities with colleagues across the organization. By honestly wrestling with this shift from the traditional role as expert to the PD role of facilitator of staff engagement, Borton and many of her management colleagues created a welcoming environment for staff from throughout the hospital to join together and make Albert Einstein Medical Center a safer place for patients. Maureen Jordon, another clinical manager at Einstein, colorfully illuminates the change in approach. "I was used to identifying a problem and getting the correction implemented, 1, 2, 3. Here's my time line, let's get this done. But then, three months later, the same problem would be happening and people would be doing things the old way. Now, it's not just me preaching. It's people feeling they have created something they own."

Sharing control and inviting ownership by the staff was an issue faced at all the Beta Site hospitals. Honest discussion about this challenging shift among peers from across the hospital members of the PD MRSA Prevention Partnership proved invaluable in making this change in orientation possible. People like Borton learned they were not alone, others were struggling too. In regular conference calls and face-to-face meetings of the members, strategies for coping with this change in role were shared, as were stories about staff contributions that emerged as a result of being invited into the process.

Other advancements in the PD process in health care resulted from the collaborative relationships developed among the eight Beta Site hospitals and their PD coaches. Many of these advancements were unplanned surprises that ended up being critically important to the success achieved by the hospitals. Among them were Discovery and Action Dialogues and new MRSA measurement systems and measures created in cooperation with CDC experts in the Partnership. These developments were outcomes of a healthy complex system at work, made possible by: regular interactions among the hospitals, participation by a diverse group of hospitals, health care professionals, and PD coaches; and the use of processes during gatherings of the Partnership that fostered creative conversations.

In Chapter 2 the statement "If the community self-discovered the solution, they were more likely to implement it" was noted as a key attribute of PD. A vivid example of self-discovery in the Einstein story is the improvs (improvisations) done around the safe transportation of patients with MRSA throughout the hospital. As you will read, many staff participated in multiple rounds of improv. These engaging learning and practice sessions helped staff witness the many opportunities for transmission, generated a myriad of improvement ideas and, over time, led to a revised hospital policy as well as a training film aptly set to the music of Pink Floyd's "We Don't Need No Education."

The Einstein patient transportation story shows that new positive deviant practices can be generated, and new policies adopted. The PD work in health care is just as much about creating new practices as it us about uncovering existing practices. As in the Einstein improv example, these new transport practices emerged from abundant interaction among diverse staff as they collaborated on a work issue. This finding is an important extension of Positive Deviance.

Chapter 6
Actions Speak Louder Than MRSA at Billings Clinic
by Arvind Singhal and Prucia Buscell

To be playful is to allow for unlimited possibility.

– James Carse

The scene is a hospital isolation room. A young patient whose gaping leg wound oozes a brown substance writhes on the bed. Her visiting mother and a nurse keep close to comfort her. A cheerfully officious doctor bustles into the room, checks the leg, blithely exchanges greetings and hand shakes with all, pats the mother on the back, and returns to the examination, bending so that a dangling necktie brushes the wound. Startling brown stains suddenly appear on everything—people, clothing and bedding. And they spread quickly from people to a surprising radius of nearby surfaces.

The ooze is chocolate pudding, a prop the Billings Clinic Improv Players use to dramatize how infectious bacteria spread through normal human contact. The actors are front line health care workers playing to an audience of their peers. Theatrically exaggerated health care hazards and the

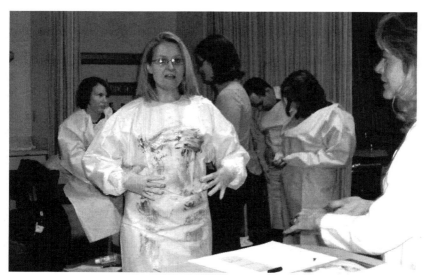

Chocolate blotches signifying infection transfer
in Billings Clinic's improv theater

goofiness of the ubiquitous chocolate blotches inspire peels of laughter. But the topic is deadly serious. And theater-style learning experiences are just one of the memorable ways Billings employees have been engaged in fighting infection.

"We know knowledge alone does not change behavior," explains Nancy Iversen, RN, director of patient safety and infection control at Billings. "We wanted to create experiences where people learn for themselves, discover solutions, and then have a safe place to practice. And we wanted it to be fun."

Fighting infection is a deep, dangerous and difficult enterprise. The microbes that cause illness and death seem endowed with disconcerting intelligence in their endless capacity for resilience and surprise. So Iversen and her colleagues found a way to shine a spotlight, at least symbolically, on the continual interplay between humans and an invisible adversary. They discovered seriously playful ways to invite everyone into the act. And in the process, they have shown that just as invisible bacterial communities can grow, adapt and flourish, human communities can communicate, collaborate and create new ways to advance health.

At Billings Clinic's 272-bed hospital, health care-associated MRSA infections declined 80 per cent house-wide since the Positive Deviance effort began in late 2006. The number of MRSA infections in the intensive care

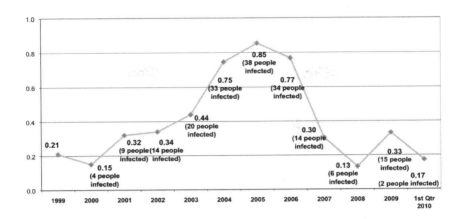

Declining rates of MRSA infections at Billings Clinic

unit, which served as the PD pilot unit, has dropped to almost zero. In 2005 and 2006 there were 28 total health care-associated MRSA infections. In the more than three years since then there have been four. Billings Clinic is one of the eight Beta Site health care systems in the PD MRSA Prevention Partnership led by Plexus Institute.

The Positive Deviance interventions focused on preventing transmission. John Jernigan, MD, MS, deputy chief of the Prevention and Response Branch in the CDC's Division of Healthcare Quality Promotion, says that's important because it prevents infection, and in addition, the epidemiology of susceptible strains of MRSA may be different from the epidemiology of resistant strains. The presence of resistant strains may be more likely to be the result of transmission. Patients infected with resistant strains are sicker and harder to treat. Further, he added, resistant strains of *staph auerus* actually may be less hardy, so if they are prevented from spreading, the overall prevalence of resistant staph is reduced relative to the strains that are susceptible to antibiotics.

"If you shut down transmission," he said, "the antibiogram gets better."

That happened early in the intervention in three of the hospitals in the PD MRSA Prevention Partnership. Declines in *staph aureus* infections were accompanied by declines in the percentage of other infections caused by the drug-resistant microbes. The antibiogram is the result of laboratory tests that determine the susceptibility of a certain pathogen to antibiotics.

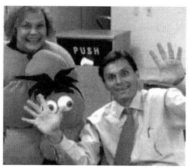 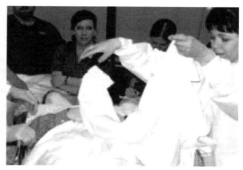

CDC's John Jernigan demonstrating his clean hands in close proximity to the "MRSA bug." Serious play was infectious.

Safe practices get serious attention as the improvisational play unfolds. A patient room is staged, and infectious disease physician, David Graham, MD, plays a 62-year-old patient with diabetes, an open leg wound, and MRSA.

"If the results of these three hospitals can be sustained and replicated," Jernigan said, "the implications are huge."

Infectious Play and New Insights

Improv theater galvanized the anti-infection effort. By acting out short dramas about keeping patients safe from infection, staff members are discovering previously unnoticed opportunities for bacteria to spread, and devising new ways to thwart the diffusion. They are also creating new conversations and new patterns of behavior that help make it habitual for everyone in the environment to follow known infection control precautions at all times. Their learning and discovery is social, visceral, kinesthetic and collaborative. And it is tailored to their own physical and social environment.

"Everyone has to be involved to stop MRSA," Iversen said. "That means changing behavior for health care providers, patients and families, and that is a challenge."

Katherine Gowan, an RN in inpatient surgical, describes the opportunities for discovery when people learn together. She remembers one improv in which a staffer said she never removed her gloves and hadn't realized she should. Another hadn't realized that it was OK to change gloves in a patient's room if they became contaminated there. "We came to realize that nothing will really change until you act your way through it," she said. "That was big."

More than 50 improv sessions have involved more than 500 Billings Clinic front line staff. The dozens of improv scenarios explored practical matters such how to clean a hospital room thoroughly, how to prepare a room for a MRSA patient, a how to transport an infected patient within the hospital,

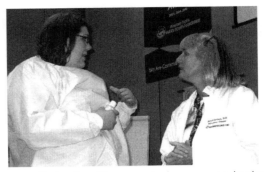

Katherine Gowan, playing a nurse in the improv theater premiere, reminds a doctor, played by a nurse, that she neglected gowning, gloving and hand hygiene on entering an isolation room. She speaks "truth to power." On-stage acting impacts off-stage behavior.

how to deal with rehab patients who are expected to be out of their rooms, how to put personal protective gear on without contaminating it, and how to take it off and dispose of it safely. Those actions sound simple, but they involve countless minute steps where possibilities for contamination abound and one small error or omission can undermine the whole purpose of infection prevention. The improvs also dealt with emotionally difficult issues—how to tell a patient about a MRSA infection, how to inform and educate families, and how to "speak truth to power"—the daunting obligation to insist that everyone, regardless of title or rank, follow infection control protocols. Hospitals are by nature hierarchical, and even experienced caregivers tend to be uncomfortable risking confrontations with physicians and executives.

The improv plays evolved with the effort to control infections using insights from complexity science and Positive Deviance as a behavior change process. The Billings approach to MRSA prevention focuses on what works, believing that among its vast pool of 3,500 employees—doctors, nursing staff, housekeepers, therapists, patient transporters, technicians, pastors, social workers, and support staff—some individuals practice uncommon behaviors that prevent microbial transmission. For instance, in doing his hospital rounds, one Billings Clinic physician purposely sees his MRSA patients last, greatly reducing the risk of transmitting the bacteria. An ICU nurse disinfects the patient's side rails several times throughout her shift to keep MRSA at bay.

The Germ of an Idea

In the summer of 2004, Billings CEO Nick Wolter, MD attended a workshop in Durham, NH, sponsored by Plexus Institute and the Harvard Center for Health Systems Improvement. Wolter was intrigued by Jerry Sternin's impromptu presentation on PD and intractable adversities. He and several hospital CEOs met with Sternin later to explore how PD might be applied to one of the most intractable problems in U.S. hospitals: adherence to hand hygiene.

When Wolter returned to Billings, he told a senior staff meeting: "This (PD) might be a 'good' idea."

"When Nick says it is a 'good' idea, it is a code word for 'let's try it'," said Jon Ness, chief operating officer of Billings. "Nick knew that when it came to hand hygiene adherence and other patient safety issues, we had plateaued with technical solutions and fixes. The fabric of leadership here is high achievement...Nick breathes quality and safety...so it was our obligation to support innovative approaches."

The importance of hand hygiene is undisputed, yet estimated compliance among most health care workers hovers around 50 per cent. Gowns, gloves, and consistent hand hygiene are often viewed as a time consuming nuisance. The Sternins' experiences using PD around the world reinforced their insight that knowledge does not change behavior. That was why Billings Clinic sought the "how" of behavior change. That "how" was Positive Deviance.

In July 2005 Nick Wolter sent Nancy Iversen to a PD workshop conducted by the Sternins in Boston. Iversen learned how people at Waterbury Hospital in Connecticut had achieved early success with using PD for medication reconciliation and she was eager to start PD at Billings Clinic

The next year, Billings Clinic helped form the PD MRSA Prevention Partnership led by Plexus Institute. In the spring of 2006 a Plexus team that included the Sternins and Keith McCandless, a principal of the Social Invention Group, came to Billings for a PD MRSA kick-off event. Staff en-

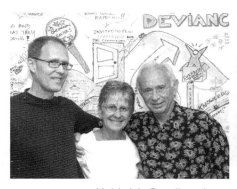
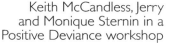
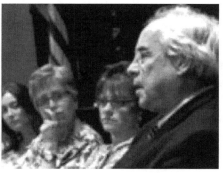

Keith McCandless, Jerry
and Monique Sternin in a
Positive Deviance workshop

Wolter, attending a MRSA Prevention
Partnership meeting with several
hospital units. He participated in key
events as the project unfolded.

thusiasm was mixed with skepticism, but the Clinic was committed to fighting MRSA, and the PD approach had Wolter's backing.

McCandless and Joelle Everett, two accomplished organizational change consultants, and Monique Sternin, were coaches for the Billings initiative. Interested staff members began meeting. In the fall, a Billings team led by Iversen visited the Veterans Administration Pittsburgh Healthcare System to see first hand the lessons it had to share. By the year's end, the Billings MRSA prevention initiative consisted of active surveillance—lab tests for MRSA bacteria—on all patients admitted to the intensive care unit, isolation and contact precautions for any patient in the hospital known to be colonized or infected with MRSA, rigorous hand hygiene, and hospital-wide use of PD processes to generate the behavior changes needed for unerring infection control in practice.

Myth Busting

The first scientific task was to get a baseline on MRSA prevalence. A study on all hospital patients and 300 volunteer health care workers in the fall of 2006 showed MRSA prevalence rates for patients were in line with national averages: just under eight per cent for patients using traditional culturing techniques, and 12 per cent using rapid testing methods. Among employees, testing showed a seven per cent overall prevalence, eight per cent among the nursing staff, and 17 per cent among physicians, nurse practitioners, and physician assistants. The licensed providers, especially male physicians, had the highest MRSA colonization rates.

It was an important step. "When we first started, there was a misconception that everyone has MRSA, I have it, others have it, so what's the point of this and why have isolation?" recalled Dania Block, RN, clinical coordinator of the ICU. "The prevalence study showed not everyone does have it."

For PD to work, everyone in the environment has to be engaged. In late 2006, coaches Monique Sternin and McCandless sat in on several focus groups with hospital staff from all services and departments to solicit their ideas for MRSA prevention and control. Participants were asked: How do you know a patient has MRSA? In your own practices, what do you do to be sure MRSA is not spread to other patients or staff? What prevents you from practicing this all the time? Is there anyone you know who has already found solutions? Soon, some staffers were beginning to provide "micro solutions" to the big infection control problems. These discussions became Discovery and Action Dialogues because the process yielded action-oriented outcomes. Still, success was not instantaneous.

"We made limited progress with DADs," said Iversen, because they often turned into "conversations that focused only on barriers without solutions."

Monique Sternin recalled, "Billings has come a long way on its own. It was not like that initially. I remember a Billings visit a few months after the launch, some time in late 2006. I was with Keith McCandless. It seemed not much had happened in those six months as far as implementing PD, as Billings was heavily involved at that time in earning its Magnet status and in conducting the MRSA prevalence study. Also, they were struggling with what PD was. I remember Keith and me sitting in a room with front line workers and the body language was telling us a lot. People had their arms crossed. Not many smiles. And someone even referred to the PD enthusiasts within Billings as the 'MRSA Gestapo.' I was telling myself *no, no, this is not what PD is about*, but it was important to not be prescriptive to those who were trying to implement PD."

Data: Disputes, Rebellion, and Inspiration to Act

"Don't be buffaloed by experts and elites. Experts often possess more data than judgment. Elites can become so inbred that they produce hemophiliacs who bleed to death as soon as they are nicked by the real world."

– Colin Powell

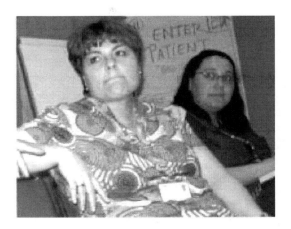

ICU nursing leaders Michaela Harakal and Dania Block at the improv premiere. "We jumped in with both feet and no life jacket."

PD depends on data. In time, the staff at Billings Clinic would become ardent measurers. But data can have unpredictable impact. The commitment to active surveillance in pilot units meant screening every single patient with a nasal swab on admission, transfer and discharge. That meant vastly more work for nursing staff and laboratory, and more records to keep. Hand hygiene and adherence to other infection control protocols would be observed and recorded, and supplies, purchases and usage would be documented. Routines would change, rhythms of the workplace would be altered, and some habits would have to be unlearned. Would it be worth it? Iversen recalls Wolter had said, "Go ahead and stir things up. We're behind you."

It was a turbulent beginning. ICU manager Michaela Harakal had been very enthusiastic initially. "We just jumped in with both feet and no life jacket, and it was my fault," she said in retrospect. "I said we have to do this in ICU. I had not thought about the impact on staff and our work processes.

"Everyone had been through staff orientation about what PD was, what MRSA was, and how we could impact it, and everyone was on board," she continued. "When the work started, and we started isolating infected patients and carriers, it threw the nurses for a loop...It was just so hard. We couldn't get all the processes down, and we couldn't get certain staff to buy into the processes of gowning and gloving."

Uncertainties, anxieties and disagreements flared. Was it necessary to put on gowns and gloves every time a person entered an isolation room to answer a call light, or check a pump? What if you didn't plan to touch the patient? Some staff

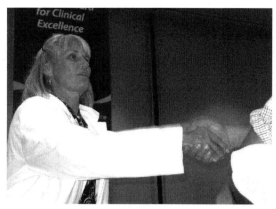

Joanie Schneider, RN, playing an un-gloved and un-gowned doctor shaking hands with a MRSA positive patient. Her neck tie unexpectedly dangled into the patient's oozing leg wound.

members wanted to find ways to avoid the gear, such as requiring it only if one crossed a line taped on the floor. "Then we had another presentation from the infection control department, showing how long bacteria can live on surfaces, how it gets all over the room, and how even if you don't touch the patient, you will touch something," Block said. "That was a turning point for us."

After nurses got past that hurdle, Harakal and Block remember working to help physicians make the same progress. "When physicians went into an isolation room without gown and gloves, the nurses wouldn't let them out until they had at least washed their hands," Harakal said. "One of our directors went into a room with gown and gloves, but didn't wash his hands on the way out. Dania is tall— 6' 1" and she just stood in the doorway with a bottle of GelSan. He looked up at her…then cleaned his hands. It was pretty funny."

Some resistance was more strident. Harakal recalls that when a nurse handed one surgeon a gown, he balled it up and threw it at her. "He was a friend of one our intensivists," she said. "I asked him to please talk to his friend and tell him that isn't something we do here."

One real indicator of success was data showing a 14-week period in the ICU with no MRSA transmissions, and admission and discharge swabbing rates that had been better than 90 per cent for months. "That gives everyone the drive to go ahead," Harakal said. "Our next step is to eradicate MRSA. We want to get to zero."

It wasn't easy to assemble the body of data that now serves to inspire action. For one thing, it takes time to gather information that shows whether something is working. As infectious disease physician Camilla Saberhagen notes, physicians like immediate results. In addition, nurses and physicians questioned the validity of the MRSA test results. Bob Merchant, MD, a pulmonary and intensive care physician, found that in the 22-bed ICU, traditional lab tests identified only eight patients with MRSA while a more expensive test identified 12. "What good are the tests, if they don't identify all cases?" he asked. The lab staff thought current tests were accurate, and demanded proof they weren't. "Never say 'prove it' to an ICU nurse," Harakal declared. "We did a two week study, and Dania saw that samples were being retrieved and sent to the lab properly, and we found that by changing culture mediums, we got more accurate results."

Paula Jackson, MT (ASCP), lead microbiologist, and her team confirmed that different tests produced varying results. After conversations with other Beta Sites and learning they were using specialized agar, she agreed to adopt this inexpensive and more specific test. But it took nearly a year to reach consensus on testing, and that was not the only issue that took time.

Many physicians remained dubious. Harakal thinks that PD is initially problematic for people accustomed to scientific, evidence-based ways of thinking. Block, who describes herself as a "true believer" now, initially thought the PD was "too touchy-feely." Many shared that view. Lu Byrd, chief nursing officer, recalls the challenge of doing active MRSA surveillance caused tensions. Swabbing all patients on admission and discharge seemed to be an elusive goal, and at one point the discharge swabbing rate dropped. "The problem was we were relying on computers to give the task to nurses," she recalls, and they weren't getting the message.

The ICU twice rebelled over data, and wanted out of the program. "We had a nice program on paper, but we weren't connecting with people the right way," Iversen said in retrospect. Weekly reports were being sent to leadership, and at one point, some transmissions had occurred, and compliance on hand hygiene and isolation precautions seemed to be down. ICU staff members took exception to the data and its interpretation. Merchant, sensing their frustration, convened a gathering to discuss whether to continue the program in ICU, and if so, how to seek commitment by all. This was at a time that many staff members still questioned whether the extra work was justified. "I was one of the people standing in front of a group saying we didn't want to do this any more," Harakal said.

Block and Harakal say doctors, including a disbelieving surgeon, are consistently using proper isolation gear now. But Block recalled, "A year ago, I'd say it was only fifty-fifty."

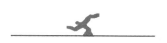

If you want to know what works, you have to ask the front line people

Tradition, Tension and Change

David Graham and Camilla Saberhagen, the infectious disease physicians, say physicians now think of gowns, gloves and isolation as requirements, not options, and that is a new attitude. But they agree physician behavior is hard to change and at first many doctors thought PD seemed irrelevant or worse. Physician education fosters and demands autonomy and independent judgment, both said. As Graham puts it, "You're put through a wringer to decide things for yourself, and if you start doubting your decisions you often become ineffective at what you're supposed to be doing."

"When you're trained in a solitary role as the ultimate decision maker, many find it harder to embrace team concepts," said Saberhagen. "When you start talking about PD, for many, that challenges the foundations of what they think of as problem solving. It's a different paradigm.

"I know some of the physicians who responded negatively when a nurse would hand them a gown and gloves," she continued, "and they are really very nice people." She adds that the PD process includes meetings, which doctors try to avoid. She and Graham hope more physicians will "come on board."

Saberhagen says her own doubts began to melt when she heard discussions among staff members who had been involved with PD. She was struck by how intense they were about helping with patient care, safety and quality. She had worked at Billings from 1999 to 2004, left, and then returned in April 2008 when the PD process was in full swing. "When I was here the first time, we were struggling with hand hygiene and isolation, and how to get it all to work," she said. "When I came back, there was a very different tone. The staff felt empowered to effect change. They were willing to speak up about what they felt was right. Many already knew what they were supposed to do. But it seemed they now really took ownership. They weren't just following rules and policies. And I think PD is the first thing I've seen that can bring about change in multiple areas by getting the right players involved. "

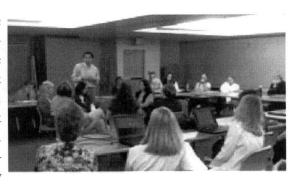

Front line nurses from several units engaged in a fishbowl conversation in the middle of a clinical leaders' council meeting. They courageously shared their observations of physician nonadherence to MRSA precautions. Pins could have been heard if they had dropped. This "fishbowl" is another improvisational way to draw out and amplify courageous conversations.

Much has been written about organizational change, Saberhagen reflects, and managers can study numbers and quality indicators. "But if you want to know what works, you have to ask the front line people," she said. "That's where the rubber meets the road. Getting things to happen on the front lines is a huge problem in health care."

Several key players remember a significant juncture that involved data, relationships and perceptions. Byrd recalls a meeting with ICU staff and leadership where she and Iversen displayed charts showing a dramatic drop in MRSA infections. Both knew the power of information made visible. A nurse asked when they could quit this unwieldy project. Upon seeing the charts, the ICU staff answered their own question: "Never."

That was in October, 2007, when the ICU leadership, Iversen and Byrd met to continue the PD MRSA discussions and try to soothe tensions. "The medical staff in that unit didn't call themselves champions—they rejected that term as a buzz word," Byrd recalled. "Pulmonary did co-develop a program with ICU. It just wasn't painless or easy."

Carlos Arce, director of organizational development, was drawn to the PD MRSA project because of its novelty and the opportunity to contribute directly to patient care. He admits he wearied of the data disputes and math wars. "Data can be used in distracting ways," he observed. "It's as though the germs have figured out that humans are inclined to argue over these figures. The departments that had the most heated arguments seemed to demonstrate the least progress. But we had to continue our work.

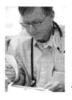

Bob Merchant, MD, examining social network analysis maps. The maps illustrated how relationships among staff were changing and growing as they worked together to fight infections.

"People look to Dr. Merchant as a leader," continued Arce. "He is an example of someone who is trusted in the organization because of how he interacts with people…We had to make sure we had healthy relationships so that we could address difficult topics and not have a defensive response. It's part of our journey around service."

John Snow and Henry Whitehead:
A Consilient Thinker and a Diligent Skeptic Tackle Cholera

In mid nineteenth century, dominant medical authorities thought diseases were caused by miasmas—poisonous, foul-smelling air arising from swamps, sewers, garbage, and the dirt and desperate conditions that accompanied urban poverty. Many more believed in supernatural causes, and rampant rumors blamed the ancient ghosts of people killed by the Plague. John Snow, a physician now viewed as the father of modern epidemiology, was interested in networks, chains of events, and ways to make the invisible visible. During an 1849 cholera outbreak in London, his analysis of the incidences and movement of disease strengthened his earlier suspicion that cholera came from something swallowed, not anything inhaled. He also noticed residents of one slum could be devastated by cholera, while those of an equally squalid adjoining area were spared, and the difference seemed to be the water supply. When cholera struck

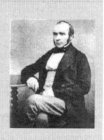

John Snow

London again in 1854, Snow created a map meticulously showing addresses of those who died in the Soho neighborhood, and found shocking numbers of fatalities clustered around the Broad Street pump.[1]

When the Board of Governors of St. James Parish—the unit of local government at the time—had an emergency meeting to discuss the outbreak, Snow presented his findings. The board wasn't convinced of Snow's water-born illness theory, but they couldn't ignore the number of deaths. They ordered the pump handle removed.

The epidemic slowed, but a death count after the outbreak showed nearly

Peggy Wharton, RN, MS, vice president of clinic operations, reflects that action can proceed in parallel with the elusive quest for unequivocal data accuracy: "Physicians will make changes if they are presented with applicable data that demonstrates the need for change. Physicians want perfection, have high standards and expect everyone to function at a high level. Data helps drive their decisions."

Lori Jens-Alran, director, medical surgical nursing, offers another insight on data and its behavioral impact. "People love facts," she said. "Then they know what's the right thing do to. It becomes black and white. We've seen CNAs (certified nursing assistants) who will hand a gown to a physician, and the physician will put it on. That's culture change."

700 people living within 250 yards of the Broad Street pump died in less than two weeks. The Broad Street pump had seemed an unlikely source of disease—its well was deep, and its water unusually cool and clear. While Snow was canvassing the neighborhood illnesses, another researcher was working separately but in parallel. Henry Whitehead was a young curate who regularly visited the sick in their homes. He began his own search for answers. He did not believe Snow's theory and set out disprove it. The Parish assembled a committee to investigate the epidemic, and invited both Snow and Whitehead to serve. Snow had written a monograph on the deaths, and Whitehead had written a detailed look at the epidemic for general audiences. While Snow had documented the drinking habits of those who died, Whitehead looked at the drinking habits of survivors. His findings convinced him Snow as right, and it was Whitehead who proved Snow's theory.[2]

Because of his intimate knowledge of the neighborhood, Whitehead knew Sarah Lewis' baby became ill at least a day before the outbreak and suffered for several days before she died. He visited Sarah Lewis again and learned she had soaked her fevered baby's soiled diapers in pails of water, which she dumped into a cesspool in the basement near the front of the house. Surveyors discovered the

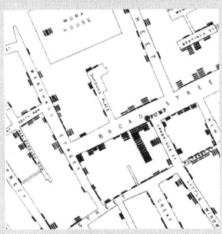

Snow used stacked bars to illustrate the numbers of the deceased, illustrating that cholera cases were centered around Broad Street pump. *Source: http://www.ph.ucla.edu/epi/snow/highressnowmap.html*

continued

Continued from previous page
cesspool was less than three feet from the outer edge of the Broad Street well, and human waste was seeping though the cesspool's decaying walls into the drinking water.

Steven Johnson, author of *The Ghost Map: The Story of London's Most Terrifying Epidemic and How it Changed Science, Cities and the Modern World,* calls the removal of the handle on the Broad Street Pump a turning point in the battle between man and microbe. For the first time, he wrote, public officials had intervened in a cholera outbreak on the basis of a scientifically sound theory of disease rather than on myth or social prejudice. It was also based on patterns of human behavior and the incidence of disease made visible on maps.[3]

While famous for his epidemiological work on cholera, Snow is also considered the founding father of anesthesiology. He is credited widely for developing drugs like chloroform and the protocols for their

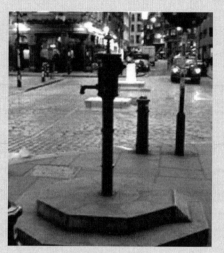

The Commemorative Pump on London's Broad Street

A Wicked Question

Life is made up of a series of judgments on insufficient data, and if we waited to run down all our doubts, it would flow past us.

– Learned Hand

Keith McCandless, who helped Billings persevere with the PD MRSA initiative, posed a "wicked question"—the kind of question that dislodges self-fulfilling prophesies: *"How is it that without complete data or evidence, we are getting great results from our prevention efforts?"*

Arce suggests some answers. One involves a Billings culture that demonstrates adaptability. Perhaps, he suggests, it has to do with Montana's western traditions of openness and a willingness to depart from convention. Perhaps it is a distant echo of the pioneering spirit that prevailed safe use. He personally administered chloroform to Queen Victoria during the births of Prince Leopold (1853) and Princess Beatrice (1857), the last two of her nine children. Johnson calls Snow a consilient thinker, whose theories were based on the connections of principles from different disciplines.[4]

Snow was a bachelor, a strict vegetarian, and an ardent teetotaler. Johnson says the reserved, scholarly Snow and Whitehead, the affable but initially skeptical curate, became close lifelong friends. Not surprisingly, Snow believed in drinking boiled water throughout his adult life.

Notes

1. UCLA School of Public Health, "John Snow—a historical giant in epidemiology. http://www.ph.ucla.edu/epi/snow.html (accessed 6-23-10); Wikipedia, "John Snow (physician)." http://en.wikipedia.org/wiki/John_Snow_(physician); John Snow, *On the Mode of Communication of Cholera.* 2nd edition, (London: John Churchill, 1855).

2. Steven Johnson, *The Ghost Map, the Story of London's Most Terrifying Epidemic and How it Changed Science, Cities and the Modern World,* (New York: Riverhead Books, 2006), 172.

3. Ibid. 162.

4. Ibid. 67. Johnson explains that the term consilience, made popular by the Harvard biologist E.O. Wilson, was originally formulated in the 1840s by the Cambridge philosopher William Whewell.

in the nineteenth century when Billings was settled as a railroad town, or the subtle influences of majestic mountains, expanses of open land and pride of place. Or perhaps it was just fierce determination.

"There is a catch 22 in the data debate," Arce mused. "Take active surveillance. If you wait until the data is in, you do nothing, and you generate no new data. Another possibility is to try everything, and see what happens to the data. I think what made us able to do that (to try everything) is a spirit of innovation, risk taking, or lack of hierarchy, and ultimately our willingness to try new things. Of course those things are intangible and impossible to measure.

"PD is rich with a different kind of data," he added. "Doing this took courage and faith, and those things can seem illogical and fuzzy. But I believe those things are what our personal *service excellence* is all about."

Personal service excellence, or PSE, as several people at the Clinic will explain, is the expectation that all staff members will be courteous and professional in all ways. They are expected to hold doors for others, address people by name and answer phones promptly. The ten-foot circle rule, for instance, requires a staff person to acknowledge anyone who comes within a 10-foot radius. A written ideal of "sharing and caring" is prominent on the wall in a main hospital thoroughfare: "We exist temporarily through what we take, but we live forever through what we give." The glass obelisk signifying Billings as a Magnet hospital, a prestigious award for nursing excellence granted by the American Nurses Credentialing Center, is displayed in the cafeteria.

The PD MRSA initiative blended well with organizational values, and some underlying changes were beginning to take root. Joanie Schneider, inpatient surgical RN, and Jennifer Mellgren-Blackford began to see increased flow of quantitative data and information about MRSA resulted in increased participation among all employee groups, and expanded infection control awareness and practice well beyond the nursing staff. "I see basic infection control practices happening in housekeeping, because people have more understanding. Nurses used to defer to doctors, and let doctors tell people about infection control. But now more people are trying and succeeding to be a part of the infection control effort," observed Schneider. Mellgren-Blackford noted unit clerks collaborated by creating new visually bolder signs for isolation and infection control in patient areas when staff noticed existing signs were unheeded. Chris Nightingale, RN, a member of the infection control team, sums up: "We encourage people to show and use what they know."

Acting, Doing, Knowing

Education is not the piling on of learning, information, data, facts, skills, or abilities—that's training or instruction—but is rather making visible what is hidden as a seed.

– Thomas More

By the spring of 2007 Iversen and her team wanted to reduce over-reliance on their expertise and encourage staff members to be responsible for infection control solutions. In earlier discussions, staff wanted a safe place to practice infection control procedures—setting up an isolation room, proper use of personal protective gear, and handling difficult conversations. As Iversen planned these sessions, Keith McCandless suggested improvisational theater as a way for staff members to explore and practice without a script, the way real life unfolds. Joelle Everett, McCandless's partner in coaching, recalled Iversen asking the difference between improv and skills competency training. She suspected skills training wasn't consistent with PD.

"It was an important turning point," Everett said. "The core team had really grasped the essential difference, and was struggling with how to implement the new way." The Billings Improvisational Theater was born. It made a reality of Jerry Sternin's saying, "It's easier to act your way into a new way of thinking than to think your way into a new way of acting."

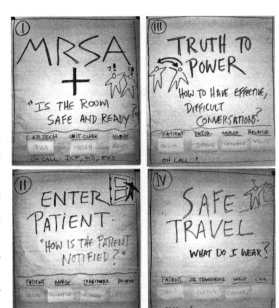

Illustrated with posters, minimum specifications for the improv scenes were drafted in 90 minutes. Themes focused on chronic challenges. New themes evolved as the improv troupe worked with different groups around the clinic.

Improv theater is rooted in Commedia dell'Arte in sixteenth century Italy. The form, with unscripted and spontaneous development of an idea or plot, has entertained world-wide audiences and in recent times has dramatized social and political goals. The Brazilian theater activist Augusto Boal created his Theater of the Oppressed so people could rehearse social action based on collective analysis of their problems. Today, a growing number of organizations and businesses use improv to improve human relationships, build new skills and find creative ways to solve problems.

At Billings, Iversen and Mellgren-Blackford made the casting calls, inviting people from different units, and worked with McCandless to envision scenarios that players would act out.

Chris Nightingale, RN, CIC, quality specialist, infection control, summarized some of the stories and insights that emerged from the MRSA improvs: "Various employees talked about their solutions for taking food trays out of rooms for patients in isolation. Some suggested the use of disposable food trays. However one employee shared her experience that if you want patients to feel unwanted, like pariahs, give them a cardboard tray with cold food. So, we didn't do that. We began brainstorming other ways to address the problem until a simple solution emerged. The nurse wipes the bottom and edges of the tray with anti-bacterial wipe and hands it to someone outside the room."

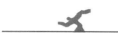

How does a front line worker remind someone more senior—an experienced nurse, a physician or an executive—to put on gown and gloves?

Workers from many units emphasized the improvs were fun, and the role-plays provided a continuous stream of 'aha' moments. In one, a nurse asked, "How does one avoid contamination if one had to hold a MRSA patient?" A colleague answered, "I put a clean blanket or a sheet between myself and the patient. It serves as an effective barrier." In another improv, a lab technician noted that MRSA can live on fabric and environmental surfaces for more than 30 days—a sobering surprise for many. In another Ms. Nightingale explained anti-bacterial hand gel is more effective against MRSA than a traditional soap and water wash. Peg Hubley, RN, infectious disease clinic office, said she always washes her own hands in front of the patients to encourage them to do the same.

The improv actors experimented with the emotional as well as the practical. One nurse told of a MRSA patient who thought he had to be isolated in the hospital because his job in a landfill made him dirty. That painful story reinforced the need for good patient education that clearly explained reasons for isolation. How do you tell a patient he or she has MRSA? Honestly, and with an emphasis that knowing the diagnosis helps with the treatment. One participant said later, "hearing how others handled this difficult conversation was very helpful. It helped me think of the right words to use to empower patients in contrast to scaring them." How does a front line worker remind someone more senior—an experienced nurse, a physician or an executive—to put on gown and gloves? The "Truth to Power" improvs offered practice. There are ways to do it politely, firmly, or perhaps nonverbally, by just standing by with supplies ready for the forgetful.

Improvs became the "in" thing. An emergency department nurse and several colleagues waited eagerly for the chance to attend.

During December 2007 and January 2008, another Billings Clinic-wide "improv festival" was launched, building on the success of the previous rounds, and learning and enjoyment were cumulative. As Jennifer Leachman, a physical

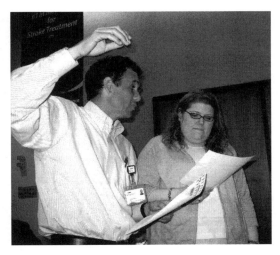

Carlos Arce serving as creative director at the premiere, starting and stopping the action. Scenes were five minutes or less with facilitated conversation between each scenario.

therapist, put it, "What one learned in one session could be passed on in the successive ones, including the precise language to convey it." Kristianne Wilson, vice president for strategic development, recalled: "The energy, momentum, and learning from the improvs kept spiraling up."

So far, only two physicians have taken part in an improv. "Don't even try," said Graham, in mock horror at the idea that physicians might be expected to participate. "You'd have a flood toward the door." He says the whole idea is too emotional and inefficient, and few physicians would see the need. Saberhagen has not participated, but she has watched, and been impressed. "I'd like doctors to watch improvs. If they could see the nurses playing the role of physicians, they would see how we are perceived, and that is very powerful," she said. "It's a view we don't often get. We don't see how nurses, other staff members, and patients perceive what we are doing." Saberhagen's observation is echoed by others who said workplace empathy was enhanced as people played in scenes that revealed unfamiliar aspects of occupations other than their own.

The nature of the improvs evolved with increasing consciousness of infection control consistency and growing theatrical finesse. At a patient safety retreat in May 2009, Billings staff members performed for an audience of 70 people, including the CEO, senior managers, physicians and nurses. They chose the skit "Truth to Power" and the title was written on a flip chart on the left of the stage area, Iversen recalls. Arce placed another chart to the right, and that one read "What makes you so special, doctor?" Matthew Kopplin, MD, chairman of the Orthopedics Department played the patient, Lu Byrd played the nurse, and improv veterans Joanie Schneider, Jennifer Leachman and Nancy Rahm completed the cast. While earlier improvs had focused on diplomacy, this performance took on a sharper tone. Rahm, playing the protective relative of a patient with MSRA, raised contentious questions—among them, she demanded to know why the nurses wore gowns, but the doctor did not.

James Reinertsen, MD, a rheumatologist and president of the Reinertsen Group in Alta, Wyoming, who had addressed the physicians earlier in the day, was captivated by the act. "It was edgy, but in a good way," he reflected later. "There is a power gradient in health care, and the rules for exception from safety and infection control go like this: Nurses always follow the rules, except when they're really busy. That's their exception, and that allows them the exemption.

"Doctors have a different version of this, and it's more about the power gradient," Reinertsen continued. "Doctors say those are great rules, but they don't apply to me. Their exception is on a personal basis, rather than on their work, and that's their exemption. The improv called out that set of things."

The scenario pointedly dramatized the impact of the "exemption" on other doctors, staff, patients and families. "When you see something acted out in front of you, and you know it isn't real—there was a little humor involved here—it still carries an important message," Reinertsen said. "You should examine from that example whether you are exempt from those rules."

Iversen and Jennifer Mellgren-Blackford remember a conversation later with physicians. Mellgren-Blackford said Kopplin reported being surprised by his own strong feelings as he played the patient: he did not want a doctor to touch him with unwashed hands. Iversen remembers a neurosurgeon saying "everyone should see this" and adding that he'd had no idea of the wake physician behavior leaves behind.

Transmitting Teamwork, Not Microbes

Live the questions now and perhaps without knowing it you will live along some day into the answers.

— Rainier Maria Rilke

Nick Wolter, the Billings CEO, reflects on the declining MRSA rates: "The recent declines are less about implementing new technical solutions…and more about improved interactions between people…Infections are being prevented at Billings by changing relationships."

Giant posters displayed at Billings in 2008 illustrated the changing nature of relationships among the 300-plus Billings employees engaged in MRSA prevention work. A baseline plot of interactional relationships in 2006 was placed alongside one from 2008.

Even to an untrained eye it was apparent that more people were having more conversations about MRSA prevention within and across units, and more cross-unit collaborations were occurring to fight MRSA.

One advantage of mapping relationships was that it led to the identification of "unlikely suspects"—people who were highly connected with others and served as a resource, but who were not previously recognized as leaders in infection prevention. One, for instance, was Sarah Leland, a young oncology nurse who emerged as a "go to person." This knowledge

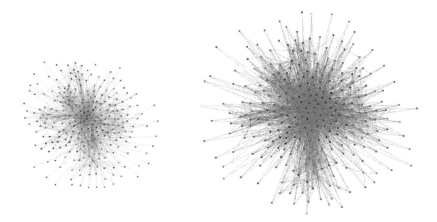

Baseline social network map before PD was implemented   Collaboration social network map 18 months after PD was implemented

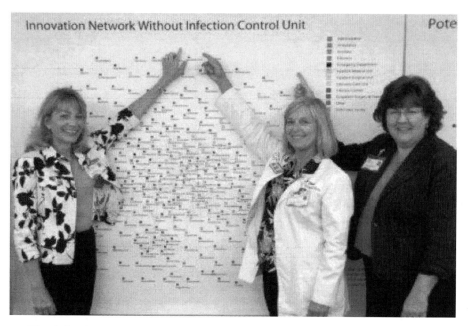

The infection control team, Nancy Iversen, Jennifer Mellgren-Blackford, and Chris Nightingale, display what a network map would look like without them. Their work in the PD initiative helped create more connections among more people working to fight infection.

allowed Clinic staff to identify people they should "especially support, draw more into the MRSA prevention initiative, and tap for influence."

The network maps visually validated that staff members who had acted together in improvs created new patterns of collaborating across units. They also enabled a sharing of collective pride when data documented success against an insidious bacterial enemy.

Ruth Senn, an LPN in inpatient surgical who played an RN and a food service worker in different improvs, says more frequent and fluid discussion among staff members brings greater understanding of what other people do and what they need in their jobs and that means more people are helping each other. "There's a PD atmosphere on our floor now," she said. "We interact as a team. We got the germ buster of the month award."

At Billings Clinic, PD and improv unleashed more direct communication among people of differing status and power. Many routine safety lapses began to be handled face to face, rather than through official channels. Courageous conversations that people prefer to avoid are acted out and explored in detail. On stage and off stage are melding.

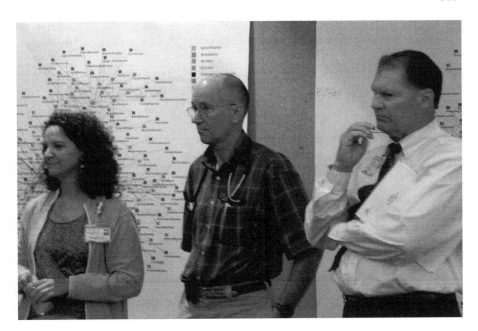

Virginia Mohl, MD, division chief for regional clinics, Walt Fairfax, MD division chief for hospital medicine, not wearing a tie and in short sleeves. Most who wear ties and full sleeves now are administrators: COO, Jon Ness.

Solutions emerged from including everyone in conversations during and after the improv. With environmental services, nurses, dietary, administration, physicians, and transport staff members actively engaged, a multitude of small changes arose. Novel solutions and unexpected camaraderie took hold along with the hope that MRSA could be stopped and lives saved. As Iversen put it, "PD is like an invitation to join a movement."

In one unexpected cultural shift, most physicians have abandoned neckties, the traditional white coats and long sleeves. As Bob Merchant explains it, some medical students cultured several neckties ties worn by physicians and discovered they harbored all kinds of microbial organisms. That highlighted the issue of clothing as a vector for transmission.

"Dr. (Walter) Fairfax stopped wearing a tie," Merchant recalls. "Ties transmit MRSA. Now the rest of us don't wear ties."

PD lets responsible managers let go of over-control and encourages eager front line staff to safely take on more responsibility. The conventional, often stereotypical, roles are overturned.

The work, and the processes that supports it, continue. Active surveillance of patients house-wide is expected to be in effect before the end of 2010. Discovery and Action Dialogues still bring unexpected issues to the surface. "We had a cool meeting recently with the environmental services team," Iversen said. "They wanted to come, and they were applauded. And we had an interesting dialogue. Some of them felt bullied. Someone would say to them, 'I need that room, you have 10 minutes to clean it.' Why would someone say that? You wouldn't want people in environmental services telling you how to start an IV, why would you tell them how to clean a room?"

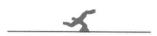

You can push for change yourself, and maybe it will sometimes work. But to have change meaningful and long lasting, everyone has to be involved and the front line staff are the people who make it happen

Delicate issues are still defused through improv. During a visit of the Joint Commission, the powerful nonprofit organization that decides whether hospitals are in compliance with federal regulations and thereby eligible for reimbursement from federal programs, a physician and nurse in radiology were observed not washing their hands after glove removal. Iversen and her team were invited to do an improv with the whole radiology team. "It wasn't voluntary, they just knew they had to do it," Iversen recalls. "They had boulders on their shoulders." Kit Hagenston, a radiology technician, challenged the hand hygiene data. She is a very high performer herself, Iversen said, and she couldn't believe others weren't. She thought improv was stupid and didn't want to be part of it. "But then she offered to act, and she did a marvelous job. She took it and sailed with it," Iversen said. "Later she thanked us and said it had been very effective. This is powerful, but it's not simple. We've seen groups change after they get started. They interact, bond, talk about how they do things. There is power in people solving problems together."

Mellgren-Blackford and Iversen say PD processes adopted in the MRSA prevention initiative have never stopped. Overall, the reduced MRSA infection rate has been sustained. But meticulous record keeping disclosed a slight increase in surgical site infections in early 2010, and showed most of those infected were previously colonized with MRSA. Iversen's col-

Confidence, With No Script and No Net

by Keith McCandless

PD and improv invite serious managers to work confidently with spontaneity and no safety net. Here are a few tips for *serious* improvisational facilitation and leadership, adapted in part from Roger Harrison, an organizational development scholar.[1]

Stay with complex questions, rather than search for quick fixes. Insights often come when we are not straining for them.

Commit to learn, to be influenced, to be personally changed—perhaps deeply and permanently—by the experience of your work.

Support a climate where speaking one's truth is welcomed, even on those occasions when doing so may make us look foolish or unprepared.

Aim for what we truly want while honoring the past and building on momentum.

We don't have to do it all ourselves. When we do our best, with goodwill, help will come. We all know what we need to know. If we have forgotten, we can help one another remember. Each person is valuable to the process. The group will invent forms of organization and work processes that suit it.

Recruit others who are willing, and at times eager, to risk doing all of the above. Often, their presence will generate unexpected solutions.

When working with volunteer improv players at the Billings Clinic, five coaching points were offered to generate more insight and novelty:

- Trust and accept all offers ("Yes, and...").

- Make action-filled choices, giving and taking.

- Engage in one conversation at a time.

- Listen, watch, and concentrate (Observe carefully, analyze less).

- Work to the top of your intelligence.

And keep in mind this insight of Roger Harrison: "I believe that all, or almost all, learning is remembering, in the sense of bringing forth what is already latent in us and giving it new form appropriate to the moment."

Notes

1. Keith McCandless draws upon several personal conversations he had with Roger Harrison in 2001.

leagues, physicians and surgeons and infectious disease specialists, began conversations inside and outside of Billings to seek solutions. One possibility under study is for every pre-surgery patient to have a spa-type full body cleaning.

Jackie Hines, director of surgical services, says PD has fostered an environment at Billings that enables leaders to value and embrace different perspectives among health care workers, and allows staff members to learn and grow with the benefit of the patient in mind.

"I have learned that ego and hierarchy sabotage health care and patient safety," she wrote in a paper, adding that she has learned answers to problems lie within her staff. She concludes, "A keen ear is needed as well as a strong voice."

While finishing her bachelor's degree at the University of Saskatchewan, Hines studied the PD MRSA work at Billings. Her professor, Colleen Vasso, who is interested in PD, encouraged her to ask questions and keep a journal as she followed the Billings infection control team during her required clinical rotation in public health. Hines says she was personally changed by the experience. "Working in the OR, (operating room) everything is drive, push, quick decision making," she said. "What I've taken away is the concept of the servant leader. You can push for change yourself, and maybe it will sometimes work. But to have change meaningful and long lasting, everyone has to be involved and the front line staff are the people who make it happen."

Editor Reflections by Curt Lindberg

Billings Clinic took "acting your way into a new way of thinking" to new heights. With limited traction gained in Discovery and Action Dialogues, leaders of the MRSA prevention effort and their coaches were searching for other ways to engage staff in uncovering and spreading good infection prevention practices consistent with the tenets of PD and the Billings culture. What emerged was improv theater, which over time reached hundreds of staff members and dealt with chronic challenges faced in keeping patients safe from infection. The improv experiences not only unearthed positive deviant practices but also helped increase participation in the hospital's MRSA initiative, got more and more staff members talking about what they could do to contribute, and provided memorable opportunities to practice PD behaviors. This, plus the inclusive, welcoming spirit of the MRSA Partnership Council and the infection control staff, led to a dramatic growth in the number of staff engaged in the PD work.

There is an important point to be made about the development of improv as a strategy for PD implementation at Billings Clinic. Each organization needs to tailor the PD process to work within its culture and this tailoring needs to be done by the people in the organization. This happened at Billings. Such refining also took place in other Beta Sites like Albert Einstein Medical Center and Hospital El Tunal as they adapted Discovery and Action Dialogues to work within their settings.

The new relationships that emerged among staff were captured in a series of social network maps shown in this chapter. They graphically illustrate the community building power of PD and the self-organizing process in complex systems. No one is in control of who gets involved and whom people choose to work with. The resulting networks are a consequence of decisions made by many people. You can say that the Billings Clinic community, using PD concepts, built the network. The increases in participation, the new relationships in the networks, and flow of information through the network are what complexity scientists have found are associated with improved emergent outcomes, which in the case of Billings Clinic were higher adherence to good infection prevention practices, lower infection rates, and an actual change in the bacterial ecology in the Clinic—*staph aureus* bacteria less resistant to antibiotics. These networks are also the highways for the spread of new practices, and what enabled the concept of social proof to play out. When one of the Billings Clinic physicians, Walter Fairfax, MD realized that ties and long sleeves could transmit bacteria, he stopped wearing ties and started wearing short sleeve shirts. Other physicians, viewing themselves as "like Dr. Fairfax," stopped wearing ties too.

Camilla Saberhagen, MD, an infectious disease physician who left Billings Clinic for a few years and returned when the PD process was in full swing, characterized these developments as involving a new sense of ownership for infection prevention among the staff.

Chapter 7
Mimes, Green Sheets and Holy Water: Infection Fighting at Hospital El Tunal and Hospital Pablo Tobon Uribe

by Narda Maria Olarte Escobar, Ismael Alberto Valderrama Márquez, Karlo Roberto Reyes Barrera, Carlos Urrea, Andrea Restrepo-Gouzy, and Curt Lindberg

Life is a series of collisions with the future;
it is not the sum of what we have been,
but what we yearn to be.

— *Jose Ortega y Gasset*

When Hospital El Tunal in Bogota, Colombia, renewed its battle against health care-acquired infections, the uniformed security guards posted at entrances to the hospital and all its nursing units began dispensing sanitizing hand gel to everyone who entered. In a decisive statement on the importance of hand hygiene, they called it "holy water."

At Hospital Pablo Tobon Uribe, in Medellin, an infection prevention campaign was lightened by the inclusion a clown's educational antics and a mime engaged to walk around the hospital dramatizing for all workers the correct details of hand hygiene. One surgeon objected to this unorthodox approach, asserting that kind of education should be "about learning at home from your mother," recalls Andrea Restrepo-Gouzy, MD. But she says most of the staff thought mimes and clowns helped make learning fun. At Pablo Tobon too, security guards became guardians of health, dispensing sanitizing gel to those entering the intensive care unit.

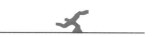

One surgeon objected to the unorthodox approach... but most of the staff thought mimes and clowns helped make learning fun.

The two Colombian hospitals serve different communities, but both used Positive Deviance (PD) in successful initiatives to reduce or eliminate MRSA infections. The front line health care staff, supported by leadership and joined by security and other ancillary workers, played vital prevention roles in both hospitals. The concept of hand gel as holy water and the ancient appeal of showmanship and humor suggest the profoundly human emotional and behavioral components of a serious professional endeavor. At both hospitals, which joined the PD MRSA Prevention Partnership as Beta Sites, the PD approach was also used to combat other health care-associated infections after successes were achieved in reducing MRSA.

Hospital Pablo Tobon Uribe is a nonprofit teaching hospital with 298 beds, two intensive care units for adults and another for infants and children, and a full range of medical and surgical services including organ transplants. Its mixed population includes the impoverished and people who use beautifully appointed reserved VIP rooms on the ninth floor of the building. El Tunal is a public hospital located in the southern section of Bogota and serves a community of 1.2 million very poor people, many of whom are among the estimated 4.9 million internally displaced Colombians forced to flee their homes to escape warring militias and armed gangs. Human rights organizations say Colombia rivals Sudan in the number of the destitute victims of relocation forced by armed conflict.[1] The hospital has 235 beds and its wide range of clinical services, which include neurosurgery and a renal unit, are intensively used.

The El Tunal Story

A 2008 issue of "Betu," El Tunal's epidemiological newsletter, reports that a high level of clinical engagement with the innovative infection control effort came about with "unexpected zeal." The whole staff participated, and eventually even hospital vendors and community members contributed to prevention efforts. Staff also created a mascot named Betu, whose image appeared on infection control materials that included T shirts, brochures, and the hospital's web site, where infection information and incidence rates are public. The name Betu itself originates with beta, and its uses illustrate the hospital's pride in becoming a PD MRSA Partnership Beta Site.

Salomon Quintero, MD, is one physician whose actions exemplify a healthy learning environment. He was the new emergency room director when the staff politely described their own infection practices and sug-

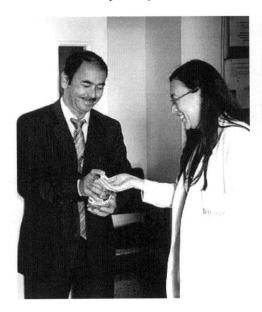

At the entrance to the neonatal intensive care unit security officer offers "holy water" to Narda Olarte, MD.

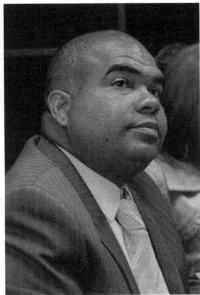

Salomon Quintero, MD, at a meeting of the hospital learning group

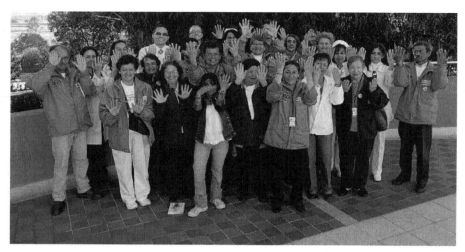

Members of the community and hospital learning team gather for a photo and give the signal for clean hands

gested he comply with them. He was so impressed with what he saw as a culture of prevention that he joined the hospital MRSA prevention learning group and eventually contributed to the community dissemination of infection control awareness. Because he also practiced at Hospital de San Jose, also in Bogota, he was able to increase the use hand sanitizers there. "Not everyone was accustomed to using alcohol-based hand sanitizer," he explained, "But…with time people are beginning to use it and I have been able to ensure that in my service it is being used in each of the units."

Hand hygiene even acquired a spiritual dimension. The gel became known as holy water at El Tunal after a guard told people entering the building that the sanitizer had been blessed by Father Chucho, a popular priest with a national TV program.

Colombian law defines health care as a public service and calls for establishment of local health associations composed of members of the community. Members of the El Tunal community organization attended learning sessions at the hospital and aided the hospital's public health goals by spreading hand hygiene knowledge and awareness in schools, day care centers and businesses. As the El Tunal newsletter asserts, "each infection we prevent means preventing human suffering, reducing risks and making better use of available funds. In other words, each infection we prevent brings us closer to a healthy society with better living conditions."

Cultural Complementary Couples

The community association used conventional instruction, but they also tapped proverbial wisdom to highlight the role of human activity in infection prevention. One familiar saying, *La gota cala la piedra*, means "the drop makes a hole in the stone." Another proverb, *La golondrina no hace el verano*, means "one swallow doesn't make a summer." By accentuating the complementary importance of individual action and collective impact, the volunteers captured the essence of the relentless vigilance needed to halt infectious illnesses.

For 10 years, El Tunal had been working to prevent health care-associated infections and to control and reduce bacterial resistance to antibiotics. The task was made more difficult by limited financial resources, crowding, inadequate physical infrastructure, and a high number of medically complex cases. In addition, staff had to address the lack of knowledge in infection control practices, individual behaviors, and the lack of a culture of prevention.

The present work focuses on hygiene, isolation precautions, education, screening patients in the adult ICU, and feedback.

Thanks to an invitation from Merck Sharp and Dohme, an interdisciplinary group from the hospital's Epidemiological Control Committee participated in a workshop about Positive Deviance and its application in public health. The workshop presentations also included work of the PD MRSA Prevention Partnership being done in six hospitals in the United States.

Given El Tunal's prevalence of MRSA and the associated morbidity and mortality, the hospital applied to join the project. Hospital El Tunal and the Hospital Pablo Tobon Uribe in Medellin were selected as Beta Sites in Colombia. This began a journey of learning and personal and institutional growth that has brought benefits already.

In October 2006 Jerry Sternin and Curt Lindberg introduced PD and shared inspiring stories of how childhood nutrition was improved in Vietnam. The infectious disease specialist of the hospital talked about the implications of MRSA for the world, the country, and Hospital El Tunal. More than 300 people from all areas of the hospital jammed into the auditorium of the public library across the street from the hospital for the first session. They included transporters, therapists, nursing assistants, bacteriologists, nurses, physicians, security guards, environmental services workers, and administrative leaders. They were joined by members of the hospital's community association—ASOTUNAL (Asociación de Usuarios del Hospital El Tunal, Users Association of Hospital El Tunal). At the end of the session, the entire hospital community was invited to volunteer in the initiative. The permanent presence of Aldemar Bautista, MD, then chief executive officer of Hospital El Tunal, fostered early success.

Tradition: A Bridge to Cultural Change

In a remote mountainous village of Pakistan, hundreds of men and women assembled in one tent with only a thin translucent curtain dividing the sexes. In a world where ancient tradition enforces strict sexual segregation, this 2004 gathering was extraordinary. The event that upset the prevailing orthodoxy was a Healthy Baby Fair, and surprisingly, the bridge between the sexes was built by honoring the culture of separation.

Monique Sternin, pioneer of Positive Deviance with her husband, the late Jerry Sternin, worked with colleagues from Save the Children to help improve infant survival in remote Pakistani villages where 25 per cent of all babies died in the first 40 days of their lives. Isolation and poverty were part of the problem, as was the tradition of strict gender segregation. Culturally, Monique Sternin explains, village men distanced themselves from feminine matters, including pregnancy. The word "birth" was considered representative of something alien, disconcerting and publicly taboo. When babies were due, women delivered in barns and cowsheds to keep the messy process of birth out of well-kept homes. Tradition and terrain maintained the isolation and insularity that made villagers suspicious of outsiders. Women, who come to their husband's villages upon marriage and rarely leave, were even more isolated than men. Pregnant women were virtually inaccessible except to their immediate families, and rarely received care from the pubic health system.[1]

All villagers had been touched by newborn deaths. They knew the problem. Sternin says the project focused on finding solutions to high newborn mortality and morbidity, and underlying gender issues were never directly confronted. Men staff members from Save the Children first approached male elders and leaders in the village and discussed the issue of infant mortality and death. Many newborns succumbed to asphyxia, hypothermia, umbilical cord and other infections, and low birth weight. The village men wanted to solve the problem. Sternin emphasizes PD helps find the solutions that already exist in communities. So the question was

Guardians Against Germs

One innovation was immediate. A group of security guards attended the voluntary meeting the day after the kick-off. After discussing the importance of hand washing, one guard observed, "We are at the entrance of every service; we can ask people to perform hand hygiene before entering the areas. After all, our job is to keep patients safe." A new PD practice was born. Guards started the practice on the pediatric and obstetrics/gynecology units, and it has spread to the entire hospital. Guards in-

asked: Do you have newborns who had survived against all odds?

Guided by male PD facilitators, volunteer men, who are more literate than the women, drew a map showing households where babies had survived, and where they had died over the last year, creating a newborn baseline. They began talking in groups about the things that happened when babies lived. In parallel groups, women—young women, mothers, traditional birth attendants, and mothers-in-law—began talking about pregnancy and births. Then men passed on their maps to the women, who made them more accurate, recording the age in months of surviving newborns, the cause of infant deaths, as well as age in months at which they died. They also added important details the men did not know. Women told of events during pregnancy, danger signs, difficult deliveries, post partum care, and things that helped newborns live. Then in both groups separately, men and women went to visit the PD families of newborns who had survived to learn what they had done differently that had contributed to their baby's survival.

Sternin said, "Most women in this culture don't initiate breast feeding for two days after birth. They would give the baby a thin drink called *ghutti* that has honey in it. But one mother in-law says she repeatedly put a newborn baby to her daughter-in-law's breast." Traditionally the newborn is laid on the cold floor, risking hypothermia. A discovered PD behavior was that homemade cushions and blankets made of discarded rags protected a newborn from a cold floor. Another traditional practice was to put *ghee*, or clarified butter, on the newly cut cord to promote healing. Actually, the ghee increased likelihood of infection. Some families whose newborn survived put nothing on the umbilical cord. Some families whose practices were different had babies who thrived.

Male villagers in their groups discovered that a husband had purchased a new razor blade and soap to prepare for the delivery. Traditionally, the husband has nothing to do with the delivery and customarily a bamboo stick is used to cut the umbilical cord. In another home visit, the volunteers discovered that a husband, unlike most others, had made plans to save

continued

Continued from previous page
money for the delivery and had secured a transport in case of obstetric emergency. These uncommon but successful practices were then shared with the larger community and vetted by the people as behaviors that they could adopt to make their newborn survive. Then the male and female volunteers designed a way to enable expectant families to learn about these and other protective behaviors that contribute to a newborn survival. They set up neighborhood meetings where the stories of newborn survival were told and where they practiced the uncommon and untraditional behaviors .

"Storytelling is so important, and people with an oral tradition are fabulous story tellers with excellent memory for details," Sternin said. Through conversation and by adopting the new behaviors, men and women in their own groups discover that fewer infections happen when the umbilical cord is cut with a clean

razor. In women's group, they made cushions and blankets out of old cloth to add to a clean delivery kit they gave pregnant women in their *mohallahs*, or neighborhoods. Newborns placed on a cushion fared better than those left on a cold floor while birth attendants delivered the mother's placenta. Separately, men and women talked about the behavior and practices that accompanied successful birth.

Husbands and wives begin talking in their homes. Men, in their groups, realized they themselves were less likely to get infections if a barber shaved their faces with

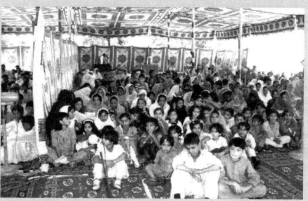

Men and women gathered at a Healthy Baby Fair in Pakistan, separated only by a translucent curtain.

vite all who enter to cleanse their hands, and they keep the dispensers filled.

The potential contribution of all groups was recognized. Security guards and high-ranking physicians shared their thoughts together, and the relationships with the hospital's community of users were strengthened. A newly created multidisciplinary learning group was trained to conduct Discovery and Action Dialogues (DADs). Under Jerry Sternin's guidance, people learned to capture the ideas of participants and help pro-a clean razor. They discovered that taking a wife to get TB shots, lightening her work load, and improving nutrition, and having a clean place for delivery led to healthier babies with better survival odds. They discussed saving money to prepare for obstetrical emergencies. Women don't leave their homes to shop, so men began buying supplies both men and women had separately agreed belonged in a kit, prepared in advance, for a successful birth. Men invited young, unmarried males in their groups, and instructed bridegrooms on their traditional Islamic duties to their future wives, including duties to a pregnant wife. That included making arrangements for an emergency vehicle should transportation be needed for emergency care.

After a few months of separate meetings, men were beginning to think about women and women's health in a different way. Villagers decided to have a *mela*, or baby fair. No babies had died for more than nine months. Fairs are usually held in colorful tents, and even traditional wedding festivities take place in separate tents for men and women. Men decided to share their mela tent with women, who would be separated only by a gauzy curtain. It was an intergenerational effort, with elders, children and families who made colorful posters to celebrate the event. Hundreds of men and women gathered, and the audience heard speakers of both genders tell stories of healthy births and thriving babies.

"We never transgressed the cultural divide," Sternin said. "It was never the plan to change communities, or change people. The PD approach takes a very specific problem, in this case the survival of newborns, and many people agree it's something they want to solve. That motivates people to change, not for the sake of change, but because of the compelling problem and the solutions they have found that already existed in their community."

Notes

1. Interview with Monique Sternin by Prucia Buscell on 5-29-10; Muhammad Shafique, Monique Sternin, and Arvind Singhal, "Will Rahima's Firstborn Survive Overwhelming Odds? Positive Deviance for Maternal and Newborn Care in Pakistan," *Positive Deviance Wisdom Series, Number 5,* Boston: Tufts University, Positive Deviance Initiative, 2010.

ponents carry them forward. Ideas, Sternin suggested, are like butterflies—to be treated gently and appreciated.

A Gracious Grinch and Scary Glitter

During a DAD on the neonatal intensive care unit, staff remembered hand cultures done during an earlier outbreak. They placed their fingers on the agar in a Petri dish and saw the bacterial growth blossom after an incubation period. They saw that microorganisms are transported on their apparently clean hands. They repeated that exercise to foster better hand hygiene practice. Today, several practices are employed with the goal of making the invisible visible. The hands of hospital

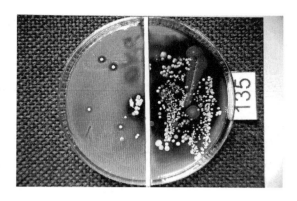

The invisible become visible in a Petri dish culture of microbes on hands before and alter hand hygiene

personnel from all areas are now cultured, and they have a chance to see dramatically different cultures from clean and unclean fingers.

The Chief of Adult Intensive Care, Ernesto Giraldo, MD, also known as "The Grinch" because he did not allow the staff to decorate the unit for Christmas, worried that the hands of the environmental services staff were dirty. He asked that their hands be cultured. His own hands were cultured as well. To his surprise, his hands showed the most bacterial growth. To everyone's delight, Giraldo gathered the environmental services staff for a party, with cake he bought, to celebrate their clean hands. He also admitted their hands had been cleaner than his. "The Grinch" then shared his story with other department heads and designated the ICU environmental services staff as the first line team in infection prevention.

Staff members created another "making the invisible visible" strategy to demonstrate bacterial transmission. Glitter was placed on surfaces such as door knobs, cafeteria utensils and coffee urns (ever present in Colombia). A team later visited the area where the glitter was scattered. Members inspected their hands, and the mechanism of microorganism transmission was dramatically visible. Since its creation the "making the invisible visible" strategy has spread to Beta Sites in the U.S.

Many members of the hospital's community association ASOTUNAL joined in the MRSA prevention effort. They met biweekly and became effective partners with the Department of Epidemiological Control, educating patients and family members. They made rounds in the hospital inviting everyone to perform hand hygiene. They also took this prevention message to community restaurants, day care centers, and schools. They disseminated information on the dangers of inappropriate antibiotic use, a valuable lesson in Colombia and other countries where antibiotics can be bought without prescriptions.

A surgeon admitted at a DAD that he had entered an isolation room without donning the necessary protective equipment. He hadn't noticed the isolation sign, displayed amidst clutter of other warning notices. He asked whether colored bed sheets might help make a patient's infection status obvious. The facilitator asked the PD follow-up question: Who else should be involved? So hospital laundry staff joined the deliberations. When color was discussed, they recommended green sheets because sheets of every other color eventually turn white in the wash. Green sheets, a new PD practice, are now used throughout the hospital as an alert to staff of the isolation status of patients.

Infection Reporting Encouraged, Data Public

After many DADs, it became obvious that people wanted positive feedback for good results and good behaviors. Several strategies were developed to recognize collaboration in infection prevention. One of the most powerful was when thirty staff members, selected by their peers for their positive deviant behaviors, received Beta Site leadership certificates presented at a ceremony by the hospital CEO and Jerry Sternin. At the end of 2008, small certificates and chocolate were given to every health care worker for achieving two months with no MRSA infections in the hospital. Hospital personnel are invited to report every infection. They receive candy or a pen for their commitment to insuring no infections go unnoticed.

Another vehicle for feedback was created by two members of the Department of Epidemiological Control. They designed an extensive set of online learning materials for the hospital staff and the public. On a public website anyone can view data on hospital infections by unit and type of infection, pictures of the hand culture results, and extensive instructional material on infection prevention practices.

During the PD work, the group learned that there are people who find solutions to problems while others find problems in the solutions. Some prevent problems to begin with. They are the ones responsible for our accomplishments and deserve recognition as unsung heroes. They save lives

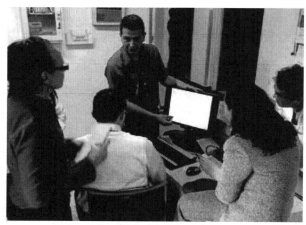

Alberto Valderama provided an overview of the intranet site developed by the infection control staff to provide information, guidance and feedback to the staff

with their behaviors day in and day out. Thanks to these individuals we can share the following results.

Since 2007 and through early 2009 the total number of health care-associated infections showed a steady decline. The greatest impact occurred in MRSA infections. Between April of 2008 and April of 2009, there were five months with zero health care-associated MRSA infections. From 2006 through 2008, the HA-MRSA rate at El Tunal dropped 59 per cent.

Chiefs of the various clinical services, who devoted time to making sense of the Beta Site experience, realized the PD skills developed by the staff and community were a special strength of the hospital and should be used to address other important quality issues.

These accomplishments did not come without difficulty. There was initial skepticism. The implementation of PD was challenging and results did not always come as expected or desired. Permanent overcrowding, very limited financial resources, and high staff turnover made it difficult to maintain consistent focus on infection prevention. After some experience the group learned to concentrate attention on those who were interested in reducing hospital infections and in using a novel method in the work.

Facilitators of DADs initially found it hard to listen to staff and not provide their own pre-conceived solutions. They struggled with some group members who did not recognize infection control problems.

Positive Deviance motivates the community to learn. Dissemination of past successes creates relatively rapid change that lasts over time. The richness of the methodology derives from the facts that infection control strategies come from peers and that colleagues realize they can follow the same strategies. Because they see the favorable impact of the changes they generate, staff members are committed to steps that help sustain the changes.

The enthusiastic and active participation by the hospital CEO, Aldemar Bautista, in early stages of the PD process proved to be of great value.

The staff plans to extend PD efforts. DADs will continue, and participants will explore how the PD methodology can be used in conversations. Other goals will be greater participation by patients and visitors in infection prevention and efforts to help the younger generation, those still in school, realize what they can do to slow development of multi-drug resistant organisms. And last, El Tunal is committed to sharing its experiences with other hospitals in Colombia.

In May 2009, Carlos Urrea, director of patient safety at Albert Einstein Medical Center, Philadelphia, and Curt Lindberg, chief learning and science officer at Plexus Institute, spent two days visiting El Tunal and talking with hospital staff and community members. They were amazed with the strength, pervasiveness and vibrancy of the infection prevention culture created by the El Tunal community. They wrote, imagine a hospital where:

- Salomon Quintero, MD, director of emergency services, was told by the staff, after observing his less than perfect infection prevention practices, "this is what we do prevent infections here, we hope you will join us." He was so impressed with the infection prevention culture that he joined the El Tunal learning group and brought the PD approach to another hospital in Bogota.

- Physicians are very engaged in the PD process. The Chief of Neurosurgery, Cesar A. Buitrago, MD, told the learning group he was proud of a nurse who reminded him to gown and glove before entering an isolation room. He commented on the vital roles played by all staff in keeping patients safe, noting that a well-done neurosurgical procedure would be worthless if a patient were not protected from infection by a myriad of hospital professionals.

- Members of the community are seen as genuine partners and experts in infection prevention.

- It is considered unethical to collect hand hygiene compliance rates in an "undercover manner" because anyone who sees another person not performing proper infection prevention is morally obligated to intervene immediately.

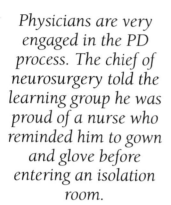

Physicians are very engaged in the PD process. The chief of neurosurgery told the learning group he was proud of a nurse who reminded him to gown and glove before entering an isolation room.

- Infection control staff members are welcomed as partners in patient care. During our visit, staff from throughout the hospital participated in the learning group meetings. When we visited nursing units, staff was delighted to see members of the infection control team and sought them out for counsel.

- Hospital staff looks to only one acceptable outcome: zero health care-associated infections. As the meeting of the learning group was coming to a close, Narda Olarte, MD asked us with clear seriousness, "What else can we do to prevent infections? Where are we failing in our PD practices?"

Well, now imagine Hospital El Tunal where hand gel is called "holy water."

Special Thanks

The authors would like to specially thank each and every one who has helped make this work posible. They include: Yaneth Arias, Adriana Serna, Víctor Sáenz, Nacira Caro, Gloria Cortes, Dolly Santoyo, Marcela Arcila, Claudia Sandoval, Diego Cubillos, Salomón Quintero, Ernesto Giraldo, Leslie Martinez, Juan José López, Gloria Galán, Martha Garzón, Carlos Mario Montoya, Elkin Lemos, Alejandro Mojica, Cecilia Pérez, Patricia Sabogal, Mauricio Páez, Fernando Gómez, Karina Jiménez, Ángela Blanco, Diana Soto, Omar Gómez y Asociación de Usuarios Hospital El Tunal (ASOTUNAL). There are many more people whose love and daily actions contribute to the prevention of infections. Even though they are not all listed above, our eternal gratitude goes out to them.

The Pablo Tobon Uribe Story

Anyone can become colonized, anyone can transmit the bacteria, so everyone is part of the problem and the solution. That realization emerged from an introductory meeting at which 405 Pablo Tobon hospital employees gathered in 2006 to learn about Positive Deviance, its use to combat MRSA, and how MRSA touches our lives.

Two MRSA patients who told their stories were soldiers between the ages of 25 and 30, both injured in wars, recalled Andrea Restrepo-Gouzy, MD. Both had chronic osteomyelitis, a bone infection usually caused by bacteria. "They were thinking where did they get this? They arrived at the conclusion by themselves that it was here at the hospital," she said. "But they were not mad. Both had very long stays here. One had one of his legs amputated, the other was walking, but with help."

Another patient, she recalls, was only a year old, and his aunt, who cared for him, began suffering from a painful skin condition. Hospital tests showed the bacteria from the aunt's skin affliction was the same as the bac-

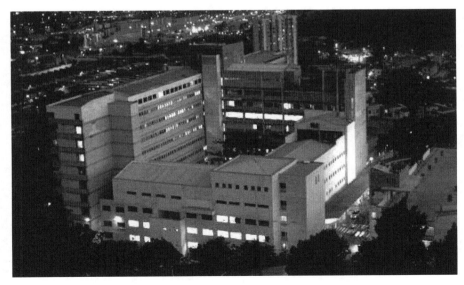

A night time view of Hospital Pablo Tobon Uribe

teria that had infected the baby. The stories of the two disabled young men, and the infected child and aunt, gave a personal dimension to the speed of bacterial spread, its devastating consequences, and the need for rigorous contact precautions.

Restrepo-Gouzy described what followed. From the first meeting a group of 45 self-selected leaders was born. The first DAD followed. Critical points were identified as necessary for MRSA prevention. They included education about known aspects of MRSA transmission and prevention, and emphasis on practices known to prevent infection—hand hygiene, contact precautions and environmental cleaning. In addition, staff discussed better communication among health care providers about infection and colonization of patients, and improved access to supplies.

Several significant new practices resulted from the dialogues:

* Dispensers for glycerinated alcohol were placed throughout the hospital, including the "Pablito" room—the play area for hospitalized children.

* Post-surgical patients in contact precautions now stay in the operating room for their anesthesia recovery. It was discovered in a DAD that when post surgery patients previously went to the recovery room, colonized and non-colonized patients were mixed together and isolation status was lost.

* Security personnel volunteered to help with hand hygiene compliance at the entrance of the intensive care unit. They remind everyone—health care providers and visitors—to perform hand hygiene.

* The intensive care unit personnel decided not to wear watches or rings at work because they interfere with hand hygiene.

* The color of the contact precautions gowns is now different for visitors and health care providers. Care providers wear blue and visitors wear green.

* Patients with MRSA infections are now assigned to single rooms.

* Patients in contact precautions get a badge placed on their gowns, indicating their isolation status, when they are taken to other areas of the hospital.

• All reusable chlorhexidine and iodine containers were disposed of. Currently only non-reusable products are used.

For the next few months all members of the infection control committee facilitated DADs with multiple disciplines including general surgery, orthopedics, radiology, intensive care, research, facilities, laboratory, and environmental services.

At the end of November 2006 the hospital had a second visit from Jerry Sternin, Curt Lindberg, David Hares, MD, from Albert Einstein Medical Center, and Jon Lloyd, MD, senior clinical advisor to Plexus Institute. In DADs with the 45 leaders, participants learned to tolerate silence, to respect and not to waste ideas, to ask people to volunteer to perform the tasks, and to make DADs fun. Restrepo-Gouzy says above all, they became passionate about the work. Hospital administration provided financial support to carry out ideas being captured in DADs.

After this visit, staff defined a new goal—zero MRSA health care-associated infections. The initial work took place in the adult intensive care unit and in a general medical-surgical unit because these two areas had the highest MRSA infection rates. The initial strategy was to focus on hand hygiene and contact precautions compliance. At this point, the hospital-wide MRSA infection rate was 0.43 per one thousand hospital days.

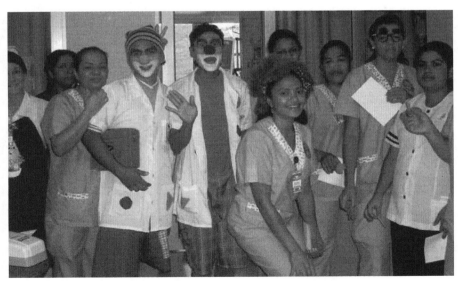

Light-hearted learning with clowns and mimes

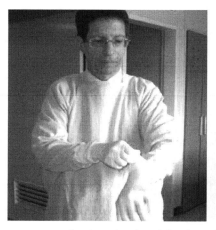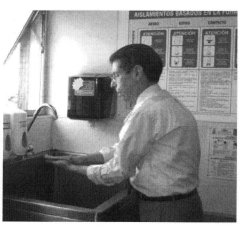

Andres Aguirre Martinez, hospital director general, sets an example

Entertaining for Safety and Citizenship

In 1995, traffic in Colombia's capital city of Bogotá was chaotic, lawless and lethal. So the newly elected mayor Antanas Mockus had 1,500 stars painted on the places where pedestrians had been killed and he hired 420 mimes to make fun of the reckless and heedless. They embarrassed oblivious drivers who ignored the black and white "Zebra stripes" painted on streets to mark pedestrian crossings, and they mimicked jaywalkers with cheerful malevolence. They helped the aged and disabled across streets, and encouraged citizens to do the same. Traffic deaths declined from 1,300 a year to 600 a year.[1]

Mockus explained his irreverent interventional style was designed to develop a culture of citizenship through experimentation and collective leadership. He also thought people would be more re-

ceptive to change if it were introduced with humor and creativity, and he believed collective social approval and disapproval are powerful motivators. In a televised interview soon after being elected, Mockus made his first splash as "Super Citizen," dressed in Spandex and a Superman cape. On national television, Mockus, as Super Citizen, jumped to tear down illegal advertisements covering the city walls. He also appeared nude on TV in the shower, giving a live demonstration of saving water by turning off the faucet while he soaped. He addressed the high murder rate by inviting citizens to exchange guns for food and flowers, and thousands did.

Mockus, a mathematician and philosopher, made visible the consequences of the careless habits of Bogota's citizens. Engaged by the non-threatening antics of street entertainers, citizens could monitor, reflect on, and self-regulate their behaviors. Further, the zany playfulness of

In February of 2007, the hand hygiene program began with the slogan "With hand hygiene we DO cure, without hand hygiene we infect." This was intentionally conceived as a program and not a campaign so it would last in time. There was a significant deployment of signs and other visual materials about hand hygiene. A mime was brought into the hospital to walk around and show health care providers how to perform hand hygiene.

A schedule for leaders was developed so they would visit all areas of the hospital and share the program with staff. Information was shared in the Hospital's news letter "En Familia" (among family), and a poster dedicated to PD was placed at the entrance of the cafeteria.

During the DADs, employee discussions disclosed contact precautions were difficult and performed incorrectly most of the time. Further, hand

the mimes provided a model for pedestrians and drivers on how to communicate disapproval of another citizens' behavior without resorting to insults or violence.[2]

Mockus' "Knights of the Zebra" campaign is another illustration of peer-regulated positive reinforcement in action. When Mockus took office, a study commissioned by his office found that taxi drivers in Bogotá were disliked and distrusted. They were notorious for flouting traffic laws, and didn't slow down or stop at pedestrian crosswalks. In an effort to restore confidence in this form of transportation, the Mockus administration asked citizens to call the mayor's office to nominate exemplary taxi drivers as part of the "Knights of the Zebra" positive recognition strategy. One hundred fifty drivers comprised the first "knighted" group, each receiving windshield stickers and small zebra figurines to display their

continued

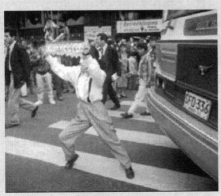

Mimes directing traffic in Bogota

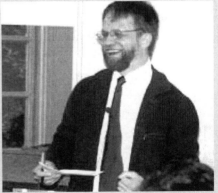

Playful Mockus

Continued from previous page
honor. Knighted taxi drivers where then invited to recruit other law-abiding colleagues and soon the "Knights of the Zebra" went from a membership of 150 to 4,800. By the end of the program, 40,000 of the 60,000 taxi drivers of Bogotá were enrolled as "Knights of the Zebra." The innovative campaign served to "make visible" the drivers' good conduct to the same citizens who once feared and avoided them.

Data collected by Mockus' office after the interventions of traffic mimes and "Knights of the Zebra" found that Bogotá experienced an 11 per cent increase in the number of pedestrians and drivers respecting bus lanes and an average of 75 per cent of drivers and pedestrians were found to be respecting the proper use of crosswalks. Mockus served two non-consecutive terms as mayor, and ran for president in 2006. In 2010, he made another unsuccessful run for president as the Green Party candidate, campaigning on a platform of social inclusion, fighting corruption and crime, and integrating the best ideas from the political left and right.

Notes

1.   A. Singhal and K.G. Greiner, "Performance activism and civic engagement through symbolic and playful actions," *Journal of Development Communication*, vol. 19 no. 2, 2008, 43-53; M.C. Caballero, "Academic Turns City into a Social Experiment: Mayor Mockus of Bogotá and his Spectacularly Applied Theory," *Harvard Gazette*, November 2004. http://www.news.harvard.edu/gazette/2004/03.11/01-mockus.html; and J. Cohen, "Calming Traffic on Bogota's Killing Streets," *Science*, vol. 319, no. 5864, 2008, 742–743.

2.   A. Mockus, *América Latina, Consensos y Paz Social*. Presentation at the 34th Congreso Internacional de Co-industria, Caracas, Venezuela. 6-30-04 Retrieved from http://conindustria.org/CONGRESO 2004/ Intervenci%C3%B3n%20 Antanas%20Mockus.pdf (accessed 6-29-10).

hygiene adherence was low despite ready access to glycerinated alcohol dispensers.

With input from many people, practical steps were designed to put on the gowns and gloves for contact precautions without getting contaminated. The hospital CEO was photographed showing how it was done and helped spread the practice by teaching others.

October 15, 2008 was the world day for hand hygiene. Two clowns were hired to spend the day walking around units reminding everyone–in a funny way–how to perform good hand hygiene.

A New Threat, Extreme Measures and Some Help from PD

Gram negative bacteria have always been a major problem at Pablo Tobon Uribe, especially *Klebsiella pneumoniae*, which infected even more people than MRSA. Gram negative bacteria do not retain violet dye used in a stain test invented by a nineteenth century scientist named Gram. Gram negative bacteria, which have outer membranes that protect the inner part of the cells, appear red or pink in a strain test. Gram positive bacteria, which include *staph* and *enterococci,* retain the violet dye. The difference helps scientists classify two different types of bacteria based on the structure of their cell walls, and those differences help decisions about treatments.[2] But because the mechanism of transmission is the same for Gram positive and Gram negative bacteria, Restrepo-Gouzy said, "We decided to focus on MRSA knowing that infections related to other organisms would also be impacted."

In January 2008 there was an outbreak of carbapenem resistant *Klebsiella pneumoniae.* Patients infected with these bacteria have few therapeutic options, high mortality, and become a reservoir of the bacteria. The outbreak may have begun with a patient from Israel who came for a transplant operation. This outbreak changed the priority of the infection control committee as well as the dynamics of many things in the hospital. For example, some entire units remained in permanent contact precautions and rectal colonization cultures for *Klebsiella pneumoniae* were performed

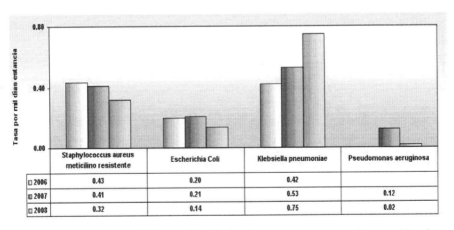

	Staphylococcus aureus meticilino resistente	Escherichia Coli	Klebsiella pneumoniae	Pseudomonas aeruginosa
2006	0.43	0.20	0.42	
2007	0.41	0.21	0.53	0.12
2008	0.32	0.14	0.75	0.02

Graph shows hospital-acquired infection rates compared by multiresistant microorganisms per 1,000 patient days. Infections from Klebsiella pneumoniae rise as infections from other dangerous pathogens fall.

every fifth day on all patients. This all took additional work and resources from health care providers and administrators. In addition, staff started to complain about allergic reactions related to the continuous use of gloves and Clorhexidine.

PD practices were used to address these issues. DADs were conducted in the five units in permanent contact precaution and positive deviants were discovered. Because hospital staff perceived the infection outbreak as a huge problem, people were eager to implement new ideas that could help. For example, nursing staff realized that certain things in the hospital were in "cleaning limbo" because no one was specifically responsible to clean them. Since then, there are always specific assignments for cleaning all the equipment. In addition, patients are assigned their own thermometers, at no extra charge. Nurses no longer go from room to room wearing protective eyeglasses, to shield them from any material that would splash during patient care, around their necks.

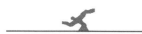

During the DADs, staff members were able to voice their frustrations and make changes to make the practices more bearable.

Some other actions that originated from these DADs include:

- Cleaning products were standardized along with cleaning procedures.

- Medical white coats with short sleeves were introduced.

- Access to isolation units was restricted to the personnel necessary to provide care. Personnel in training were not allowed inside.

- Unnecessary objects were banned from the intensive care unit.

- Medicated hand lotion was provided to staff to prevent contact dermatitis related to gloves and hand hygiene.

During the outbreak, many extreme measures were necessary, such as closing beds, assigning infected patients to cohorts and certain health care providers, and the use of scrubs was required in all units in isolation. (In March 2009 the CDC recommended that all U.S. patients infected or colonized with carbapenem resistant *Klebsiella pneumoniae* be placed on contact precaution.) These measures were essential for the control of the outbreak but at the same time were very inconvenient for staff. During the DADs staff members were able to voice their frustrations and make changes to make the practices more bearable. A coffee room with small rest area was installed for staff who had to spend their entire shifts, without leaving or returning, in the area designated for *Klebsiella* patients.

Persist, Resist, Do Not Desist

"Positive Deviance has allowed us to get closer to people to solve problems together, and we have learned that within the problem is the solution," Restrepo-Gouzy observed. The MRSA infection rate decreased to 0.32 per one thousand patient days, and, as expected, infections related to other microorganisms have also decreased. PD has also been helpful to control the outbreak of *Klebsiella pneumoniae*

The MRSA infection rate decreased to 0.32 per one thousand patient days, and, as expected, infections related to other microorganisms have also decreased.

Since 2006 there has been a trend towards the reduction of the overall hospital infection rate from 6.2 to 4.4 per one thousand hospital days. "This effort has resulted in a different hospital culture," she said. "We believe there is a more positive and conscious attitude regarding hand hygiene. There is also a better knowledge about the transmission and prevention of hospital-acquired infections. This is reflected in the improved compliance for hand hygiene and contact precautions."

"But not everything has been easy; we have found some obstacles along the way. HPTU is a hospital with very complex cases and with established protocols for almost everything. That makes change difficult," she said. "We have also encountered negative deviants who put barriers to the ideas of others. Health care providers are busy and it is difficult to find the time for DADs. However, this has taught us that in order to prevent infections you have to persist, resist, and not desist.

"And finally, in addition to helping us reduce hospital-acquired infections, Positive Deviance allowed us to meet highly valuable and interesting people: Jerry Sternin, Curt Lindberg, Henri Lipmanowicz, Jon Lloyd, and David Hares. To them goes our eternal gratitude for believing in our country and in our hospital. Jerry's legacy will remain in our hearts. We will remember him as a friend who taught us to face our problems in a positive manner and to see in each idea the enormity of the human being."

Special Thanks

The Infection Prevention Committee wants to acknowledge all the people that made possible the Positive Deviance initiative at the Hospital Pablo Tobón Uribe. To name all the people involved who contributed to the project would be impossible, but they include everybody from the Chiefs of Staff, administration, health care staff and ancillary services. We would like to thank our patients and their families for allowing us to learn from their experiences. We also want to make a special mention to Merck Sharp and Dohme Laboratories for their financial and logistic support, which was essential for this learning experience.

Endnotes

1. Norwegian Refugee Council, Internally Displaced People (IDPs) in Colombia, "New Displacement Continues, Response Still Ineffective," Internal Displacement Monitoring Centre. http://www.internal-displacement.org/countries/colombia (accessed 5-25-10).

2. Maryn McKenna, *Superbug: The Fatal Menace of MRSA*, (New York: Simon and Schuster, 2010), 182.

Editor Reflections by Curt Lindberg

The involvement of "unusual suspects"—those not typically involved by hospitals in solving a clinical dilemma—is one of the strong themes in the stories of the two Colombian hospitals recounted here. Security guards adopted an expanded definition of their security duties by offering to dispense hand gel to everyone who entered nursing units. "After all," one guard said, "our job is to keep patients safe." After an embarrassing episode for the physician director of intensive care at Hospital El Tunal, he declared the environmental service workers the "first line team in infection prevention." The expertise of laundry staff was tapped in a decision about what color linen to use to signal the isolation status of patients.

El Tunal even reached outside the hospital to involve unusual suspects—residents of the hospital neighborhood. These neighbors became extensions of the hospital's infection prevention and infectious disease staff by staying alert to infection trends in the community, talking to patients about the importance of hand hygiene, and educating friends and family members about how to prevent the spread of antibiotic resistant bacteria.

As noted in Chapter 3, when change is sought diversity is your ally. The different perspectives and experiences brought by unusual suspects and welcomed in the PD process certainly helped fuel the advances in infection prevention in these two institutions.

When the two Colombian hospitals came to appreciate the importance of "bathing" the PD process in data, they thought expansively. At Hospital Pablo Tobon Uribe they invited two soldiers who had contracted MRSA in the hospital while undergoing treatment for war injuries to tell their stories to hundreds of staff members who attended the MRSA prevention kick-off meetings. At Hospital El Tunal the hands of staff members were cultured for MRSA and the results were posted, without reference to individual workers, for all to see on the hospital's website. Also on this website, which is public, are more regular types of data like infection rates by unit. In addition, glitter, placed on door knobs and coffee urns, helped staff appreciate how easy it is for invisible substances to spread around the facility on the hands of health care workers.

Another important contribution from the PD work in health care was the extension of PD to another serious patient safety problem—controlling an outbreak of a carbapenem resistant *Klebsiella pneumoniae* at Hospital Pablo Tobon Uribe. With experience gained using PD for MRSA prevention, leaders of infection prevention had the confidence to use the process to help staff deal with this deadly antibiotic resistant bacterium. This development extends the application spectrum of PD from medication reconciliation, to MRSA, and now *Klebsiella pneunomiae*, building the case for its relevance to many complex patient safety and quality challenges.

Chapter 8
Positive Deviance:
Success in Human Terms
by Margaret Toth, Sharon Benjamin, and Joelle Lyons Everett

The pattern . . . is there from the start. Your task in life is to discern that pattern, listen for it, and give room for it to emerge.

> — *Roger Housden*

"While observing hand hygiene practices on one of the nursing units, I saw our Jasper arrive to transport a patient. He was a bit down the hall from me but I could hear him talking to a patient care assistant in a room across the hall who had just disposed of an isolation gown, a bit sloppy for Jasper's liking I guess. I could hear him saying 'There's a way to do that so there is not so much trash.'

"After hearing him explain, she said 'I don't understand.'
With that, he took a short break from his duties and
grabbed an isolation gown saying, 'OK, isolation gown removal, here we go' and proceeded to demonstrate his
'method' right there in the hallway."

> *Catherine Reynolds, RN, MJ, DL*
> *Quality Improvement Coordinator*
> *Albert Einstein Medical Center*
> *In-house Facilitator*

A lmost unimaginable. In 2005 at least 20 people, whose recoveries were
a statistical surprise, left Albert Einstein Medical Center and returned
to their lives and families. Only a year earlier (or if hospitalized at perhaps
a thousand other US hospitals) the odds dictate that this same number of
patients would have acquired a disabling health care-associated infection.

How did this health care community transform into one where Cather-
ine Reynolds can observe broad-based ownership and effortless cooperation between previously distinct staff silos? How did this manager come to
experience not only the obvious reward of improved outcomes, but the
exhilarating satisfaction associated with an earnest, cooperative and joyful
workplace? How did she come to terms with her new role as a catalyst
rather than workhorse for change?

One of the answers for this hospital, along with the other health care
organizations discussed in this volume, has been the use of Positive Deviance (PD). But this is an extremely difficult approach for managers,
change agents and consulting coaches to apply. It humbles, disrupts, un-
nerves and burdens in-house facilitators and the external coaches who
support the process. As a result, PD is rarely embraced when alternative
and more conventional approaches seem promising. Best practice and
lean/six sigma inspired approaches are easily accepted and carry less professional risk. Thus, it has been said that PD is most suited for people and
communities that have exhausted these other options and turn to PD desperate and frustrated.

The aim of this chapter is to peek into the world of managers and
coaches who have plunged into PD and formulate a reflective and perhaps
persuasive case for using Positive Deviance before all else fails. We'll highlight some of the reasons PD seems to be particularly effective in address-

ing complex challenges: engaging everyone; honoring the local culture; inviting volunteers to join the effort; and using locally developed data to drive the process.

For this chapter, we interviewed the coaches and hospital staff who pioneered the use of PD in health care. In retrospect, we can identify the elements of their journey that contributed to success or halted progress. But in reality, each journey was messy and the outcomes not assured. In retelling their experiences, the coaches and hospital staff offered an unvarnished assessment of their experiences, doubts, surprises, and insights.

Introducing Positive Deviance in the Hospitals

Engaging Hospital Leaders

For the hospitals involved in the Positive Deviance pilot, the *introduction* began long before many of the in-house facilitators and managers became involved. A loosely connected network of health care quality improvement leaders, hospital executives and the complexity innovators associated with Plexus Institute learned about Positive Deviance from its founders, Jerry and Monique Sternin, and Tony Cusano, MD, the physician who pioneered the use of PD at Waterbury Hospital in Connecticut.

Hospital senior leaders were exposed to both the *concept* of Positive Deviance (the fact that in every community, no matter how disadvantaged, some people, with access to no more resources, will have superior outcomes) and the PD *approach*, the behavior change approach created by the Sternins to capitalize on these in situ successes. These leaders responded positively to the inherent economy of the approach (amplifying existing practices), the track record of their relationships within the network and the opportunity to be among a select group of facilities pioneering the PD approach in health care.

New Coaching Roles: Anticipation and Anxiety

With an invitation from the hospital leaders, PD coaches from Plexus and hospital staff identified by senior leaders to become in-house facilitators formed a working partnership. For both the PD coaches and the hospital staff, introducing Positive Deviance was unsettling. Both excelled as problem solvers and technical experts. They were familiar with other improvement approaches and yet had to simultaneously translate and learn a new approach, while dramatically altering their own behavior and role. A combination of gnawing skepticism and great anticipation characterized their real-time experience.

Everyone Into the Talent Pool

For physician leaders, quality managers, and infection preventionists who were in-house facilitators, the open-ended introduction of PD deviated from standard practice. Instead of presenting a small group of representative staff with PowerPoint slides neatly outlining a project vision and mission statement, clear change practices and marching orders, PD was introduced to all comers at a kick-off with stories about combating malnutrition in Vietnam and an invitation for those with an interest in using a similar strategy to combat health care-associated MRSA infections to return as volunteers.

Engaging More Staff by Improving Our Invitations

One of the questions that comes up repeatedly in our conversations about preventing MRSA is, *"How do I engage more staff in MRSA prevention?"*

And, that's a great question because how we invite people to join us—that is, how we evoke true, sustainable engagement-- always starts with our invitations.

Peter Block, a well-known organizational change consultant, often says: "All we have to offer is our invitation." By this, he means that we can fool ourselves into believing that we can cajole, or even coerce, people into becoming engaged. But really, only sincere, attractive invitations actually result in real engagement.

So, what makes an invitation to become involved irresistible? Here are some strategies used by in-house facilitators to encourage staff to attend PD "kick-off" sessions.

* *Invitations offer authentic hospitality.* Great invitations let people know that they will be treated with generous and cordial consideration. Their needs will be attended to and their contributions will be valued.

* *Great invitations are personal.* Aren't we all flattered when someone we respect and like asks us to join them for a fun and important event?

* *The invitation is attractive.* Invitations don't necessarily have to be for "fun," but tempting invitations do have to

"It seems risky talking in an abstract manner in an evidence-based medical environment. You risk your own credibility—it's a big risk."

Kay Lloyd, FACHE, Vice President,
Operations Improvement, University of Louisville Hospital,
In-house Facilitator

"When we introduced PD to our peers, it was not immediately obvious this will work. We heard, 'show me the money,' and we did not have the proof originally."

Wendy Ziai, MD, Assistant Professor of Neurology, Neurosurgery,
and Anesthesiology and Critical Care Medicine, The Johns
Hopkins Hospital, In-house Facilitator

appeal to the interests and needs of potential guests.

- *Tempting invitations make it easy for people to say yes.* We'll have more success engaging people when we invite people for shorter rather than longer durations and when we ask them to join us in a convenient location (which often means that we go to them instead of asking them to come to us!).

- *The focus of the invitation is about building a better future.* Habitat for Humanity recruits thousands and thousands of volunteers to come create a better future for people who need housing. Notice that Habitat does not invite volunteers to come and get tired, hot and dirty hammering nails. The result? Habitat has built more than 250,000 houses around the world, providing more than 1 million people in more than 3,000 communities with safe, decent, affordable shelter.

- *Appealing invitations are specific* about why the person is being invited, what they can contribute and when the event will start and end and where it will be.

- *There's a promise of both the familiar and something exciting.* It's hard to get people excited about "the same old same old" and it's hard to get people to adventure into the completely unknown. Good invitations offer just enough familiarity to feel safe with a big enough dollop of novelty to be enticing and entertaining.

The first act for in-house facilitators was to orchestrate the loosely scripted gathering of the hospital community referred to as a "kick-off." The primary purpose of the kick-off was to communicate that this was not going to be another typical improvement initiative.

> "One of the biggest shifts for facilitators was realizing that their role was not to tell staff WHAT to do but to figure out HOW they could create an environment for the staff to figure out for themselves what they already do and what they might do. It's hard because for the managers it feels like they are not doing their job. They are paid to solve problems. To make matters worse, if they are really good at creating space for others to solve their problems, it looks like they are not doing anything. Of course, that is not true at all; it takes a ton of work but it's invisible."
>
> *Margaret Toth, MD, PD Coach*

> "It was risky to invite participation and truly give people the opportunity to opt in/opt out at every level of the initiative. In the Beta Sites what happened was revolutionary—the teams that formed were self-selected and volunteer—the work that was carried forward was carried by staff who volunteered. No overtime pay, no coercion, just a question: 'If you think this is important, what will you do to help?'"
>
> *Sharon Benjamin, PhD , PD Coach*

During the planning and execution of the kick-off, the role of the PD coaches was to guide in-house facilitators to avoid slipping back into an authoritative, expert stance. In PD, the highest level of expertise belongs to the individuals whose behaviors must change if a problem is to be solved. In hospitals these people were those whose "touch" put them in contact with germs that could harm patients. The notion that housekeepers, hos-

Eliminating the Transmission of MRSA Infections
by Using Positive Deviance (PD) Approach to Behavior and Social Change
May 10 & 11, 2006
AGENDA

PRE-PLANNING SESSION: Wednesday, May 10th, 2006

0900 – 1100	Review of Meeting Plan & Session Objectives (PD/MRSA Planning Team)
1100 – 1200	Lunch PD/MRSA (Planning Team)

SESSION I & II: May 10 & 11, 2006

1300 – 1315	Welcome & Introductions (Mark Rumans, MD)
	• MRSA is an imperative patient safety issue that needs addressing & why Billings Clinic is uniquely positioned
	• Billings Clinic selected as a Beta SitE
1315 – 1400	Background (Ed Septimus, MD, Nancy Iversen, RN, CIC)
	• Brief history of MRSA in US and at Billings Clinic
	• The Billings Clinic Story – The Human Face of MRSA Infections
	• 3 Stories – Patient, Surgeon, Family Member perspectives
1400 – 1500	Introduction to Positive Deviance (Plexus Institute Faculty
1500 – 1515	Break
1515 – 1600	Group Exercise – Case Study (Plexus Institute Faculty)
1600 – 1615	Reflection of the Day (Plexus Institute Faculty)
1615 – 1630	Invitation to join core group and next steps (Plexus Institute Faculty)

Billings Clinic kick-off meeting agenda

pital volunteers, security guards, medical assistants, doctors and staff nurses know more about preventing infections in their areas than infection preventionists and quality managers runs counter to accepted beliefs. PD coaches improved the in-house team's first experience drawing out staff expertise during the kick-offs by prompting them to include generous blocks of time for reflection and audience interaction, arranging seating to avoid classroom configurations, soliciting local stories, and learning to wait patiently for staff to respond to questions.

Inspiration from the Founders of PD

Before successful experiences with PD and MRSA prevention existed, the hands-on field experience in PD, such as that offered by Jerry and Monique Sternin, provided facilitators with powerful validation for this uncommon approach. As PD coaches, Jerry and Monique modeled, at every turn, the very behavior they asked facilitators to try. In each of their stories and interactions Jerry and Monique demonstrated supreme respect for the intentions and culture they described in their examples. Jerry and Monique's deep, authentic deference to local culture helped disarm suspicions and defensiveness that any new audience might be expected to harbor towards outsiders.

Introducing PD into the participating hospitals by telling, and deconstructing, the PD story in Viet Nam was bolstered by Jerry and Monique's credibility—taken together, the story and the personalities were powerful motivators. Talking about PD became a jumping off point for members of the community accepting the invitation to volunteer and move to action. Thus, like many risky journeys to new lands, having Jerry and Monique serve as the initial, experienced guides was powerful and seemed essential. Now, however, as others have gained experience with PD and learned from Jerry and Monique, the voice of experience for PD comes from a larger community and kick-offs have been successfully replicated without need for the PD founders' presence.

Senior Leaders Speak and Listen

Ultimately, for in-house facilitators, the response of those positioned above and below them in the hierarchy eased the introduction of PD. In each hospital, the decision to try the PD approach was made by its most senior leaders. Frequently board members, senior executives, PD coaches and in-house leaders celebrated this invitation with a reception the evening prior to the launch of the PD approach. Hospital CEOs were consistent in making public their tacit confidence in the PD approach, despite the absence of a predetermined path.

> "I don't know what this will look like, but the staff will know."
>
> *Rajiv Jain, MD, Chief of Staff,*
> *VA Pittsburgh Healthcare System, Senior Leader*

The hospital staff, in turn, demonstrated their willingness to accept this role change among managers through their enthusiastic response. As

attendance at kick-offs exceeded expectations and 50 or so attendees returned as volunteers, in-house facilitating teams' confidence was bolstered.

> "We wondered, are we wasting time with something un-
> proven? After the first encounter, we were amazed by the
> level of engagement. It was a hard-core bunch. They were
> engaged. We heard people say, 'They cared what we said.'
> Past that, there was no more risk. Well, maybe some risk
> when we went to the executive committee. But that turned
> out to be just as engaging. It was good learning. Not a cog-
> nitive issue, but part of the affective domain."
>
> *Patricia Norstrand MS, RN BC, Senior Director,*
> *Department of Quality, Risk and Safety,*
> *Franklin Square Hospital Center, In-house Facilitator*

The Early Stages—Starting Small to Move Fast

The pressures in-house facilitators faced in combating health care-associated MRSA infections were substantial. Not only were lives at risk, but
hospital accreditation and reimbursement rates were increasingly linked to
reducing infection rates. Allowing the open-ended PD change approach to
take hold at its own pace became especially difficult because the start of PD
appeared to be slow and small in scale.

Igniting Social Proof

In PD the action starts small and local for a reason. This is not to get
early success to roll out and replicate, but rather what is sought are early
successes. These successes build the social proof and thus the credibility
that great ideas already exist and can rapidly ignite and spread through existing formal and informal hospital networks because they belong to staff
and already work in the context of their unique circumstances.

Discovery and Action Dialogues Uncover Real and Potential Successes

Following the initial excitement of kick-offs, efforts to uncover positive deviant practices as well as the more common latent practices (good
ideas staff had but never acted on) were carried out. A common approach
involved smaller gatherings of staff—sometimes lasting no more than 15

or 20 minutes, during which in-house teams facilitated Discovery and Action Dialogues (DADs). Although many hospitals had experience discussing problems with staff, the nature of the PD questions created more open and generative conversations. At times, the very success of these lively sessions halted the PD process as in-house facilitators, anxious to accelerate change, unintentionally took over staff ideas and took over responsibility for their follow-through. Facilitators quickly became bottlenecks and limited the number of discovery sessions based on their own limited time, energy and competing priorities.

Strategies PD coaches used to anticipate this outcome included periodically re-training in-house facilitators to capture positive deviant behaviors and return them to the communities for action. The coaches also emphasized the overriding importance of reaching hundreds and thousands of staff through discovery sessions over a shorter period of time. By stressing the need to engage a substantial proportion of the staff, the in-house facilitators were forced to give back the ideas that accumulated quickly and exceeded their own capacity to act.

In-house facilitators often worried about staff participation in DADs, yet they were received with nearly universal enthusiasm. PD coaches emphasized skill building for the in-house facilitators, using fishbowl exercises and having teams of in-house facilitators immediately practice with groups of hospital staff. In-house facilitators found it useful to work in pairs, take

> **Guiding Questions for PD Discovery and Action sessions**
>
> - How do you know whether your patient has MRSA or carries the MRSA germ?
>
> - In your own practice, what do you do to prevent spreading MRSA to other patients or staff?
>
> - What prevents you from doing these things all the time?
>
> - Are there any individuals or groups that have a way of doing things that helps them overcome these barriers?
>
> - Do you have any ideas?
>
> - What would it take to make any of these ideas happen here? Any volunteers?

Guiding questions for PD Discovery and Action Dialogues

time to debrief among themselves afterwards, and modify their guiding questions in a way that felt most genuine and natural to them.

We asked the University of Louisville team, "Were you using the guiding questions at first?"

> "Our process was pretty messy. When our coaches were there it went much better. It became easier, especially with the dialogue sheet they gave us. With our coach we walked all over the place, every part of the hospital. We asked questions, tried to model discovery and action. We walked with night shift, day shift, lots of people."
>
> *Linda Goss, ARNP,*
> *Director, Infection Control and Vascular Access Nurses, University*
> *of Louisville Hospital, In-house Facilitator*

> "People feel respected and their input is valued. Other initiatives stifle creativity. We have seen so much creativity, from unlikely sources."
>
> *Nancy Iversen, RN, CIC, Director of Patient Safety*
> *and Infection Control, Billings Clinic, In-house Facilitator*

PD Inquiry–Hospital Innovations

The PD coaches observed liberating innovations when the in-house staff was pressured to reach as many people as possible. Billings Clinic used improvisational theater (improv) during orientation and yearly in-service to reenact common patient care scenarios. Franklin Square Hospital Center vastly increased its capacity by training volunteers to fan out across the health system and conduct discovery and action sessions.

While meeting with large numbers of staff early on felt like a slog, and created a slow start, it laid the groundwork for the exponential improvement typical in PD applications. Supportive guidance and confidence offered by PD coaches proved to be an essential contribution at this stage.

Improv turned out, at Billings, to be a fun and engaging way to do discovery and action. Many of the challenges in a hospital take place in a social and interactive setting, and by playing out a scene, the players could explore the situation interactively and kinesthetically, and experiment with different solutions. The audience could see the small details of an isolation precaution or a difficult conversation, and try out new ideas they observed. The discovery and action questions were incorporated into debrief sessions after the scene. Coach Joelle Everett was in the audience for the debut of the Billings Players, a group of volunteers from the Prevention Partnership council that used this method to teach hand hygiene and isolation precautions throughout the hospital.

> "There were probably 40 people in the circle, and the body language in the room was amazing. Everyone was leaning forward, following the action, taking notes, and laughing. How often do people leave a meeting and tell their friends how much fun it was? We were astonished when we read the debrief sheets. People had learned so much in less than one hour."
>
> *Joelle Everett, MS, PD Coach*

Data: Part of the How

Like all good process improvement approaches, PD is bathed in data—from outcomes data to process metrics, data sat at the center of the MRSA efforts. In fact, one of the great contributions Jerry and Monique Sternin made to behavior change was trusting that it was almost inevitable that PD practices and behaviors would exist, and recognizing that it was essential to turn the data in which this was embedded over to the community—be it a village or hospital—to discover, and over time use it to monitor for progress. This is a part of the *how* that makes the PD approach work.

The Challenges of Data

Getting outcomes data (MRSA transmission and unit specific infection rates) to establish the impact of the PD approach was hard and slow work everywhere. And it was essential. With the science and evidence-based mindset in the hospitals, outcomes data are needed to demonstrate that MRSA is a problem that should be addressed, and that changing individual behavior can make a difference. The PD approach is only useful when the community believes there is a problem. Having these data and presenting them to the community so they can identify the problem rapidly disarms denial.

With tens of thousands of patients moving through a typical hospital, gathering data regarding MRSA carriage, transmission, and outcomes is complex and often overwhelms existing data retrieval capacity and human resources. "Data was horrendous," Norstrand recalled. "We could not get what we needed. I wish we were starting over. If we were beginning now, it would be different. Lack of data clouded the process. We did not have the numbers."

Several issues conspired to make data collection on outcomes difficult. Gathering active surveillance data (identifying MRSA transmissions by collecting nasal cultures from each hospital patient at admission, transfer and discharge) was non-existent at all but a handful of hospitals and required senior leadership sanction as an unreimbursed addition to patient care costs. Once the decision to collect these data was made, putting in place protocols for charting orders, collecting specimens, increasing laboratory capacity, tracking and analyzing results and informing patients became time consuming and competed with PD implementation itself.

Early on the hospitals decided to develop a consistent system for reporting data so they could compare results in a meaningful way. Hospital epidemiologists and infection preventionists worked cooperatively with the Centers for Disease Control and Prevention (CDC) to enhance and test a module developed for the National Healthcare Safety Network (NHSN) reporting system.

Information Wanted, Right Here, Right Now
While tremendous improvement occurred despite the absence of outcomes data, both in-house facilitators and coaches agreed that the PD initiative would have been more robust and perhaps accelerated if these data were available at the start of the intervention.

One reason the absence of hospital-level outcomes data did not prevent progress was because in-house teams were able to generate more vital local data. An early demonstration of this occurred at The Johns Hopkins Hospital. Ziai had invited staff from the Neurosciences Critical Care Unit (NCCU) to discuss the health care-associated infections. She sat among a group of busy nurses, receptionists, medical assistants and physicians stealing a few minutes of their time in a crowded, warm conference room with a small packet of graphs in her hand. She passed around the packets and quietly asked the hurried group—critical by nature—to look at it with her. The hospital's epidemiology department had quietly collected environmental cultures from rooms that had been cleaned after patient discharge. Together the group discovered that the "clean" rooms harbored dangerous germs. Sharing these data, and not the interpretation or action plan, triggered a pattern of cooperative and dispersed problem solving that transformed the NCCU staff and sharply reduced its infection transmissions.

Similarly, when Kay Lloyd took data to a staff meeting and went over it, she said "I got lots of questions, 'why' questions. I thought *wow, they really want more information! It evoked a hunger in the staff." She saw that PD is only useful when the community believes there is a problem, and immersing the groups in their own data led to introspection and quickly dissolved common "lack of evidence" and "inevitability" deflections.

Making Data Personally Relevant

Another function of data in the PD approach involved reinforcing the breadth of the health care infection problem. The hospital staff in the Beta Sites shared the frustration common to professionals facing the difficult problem of health care-associated infections. For years, health care infection rates had been published. Hand hygiene campaigns came and went. Progress was hard to maintain, and burgeoning drug resistant organisms were making the challenges increasingly complex. Changing external forces, such as threats of reduced reimbursement and increased regulatory scrutiny intensified the need for innovative action. In addition, a renewed effort had to make infection prevention seem vitally important to members of a diverse hospital community that would include janitors, food service employees, nurses, doctors, executives, patients, and volunteers.

The problem became meaningful—when it was reframed by the staff. Abstract numbers became personal stories—often involving health care workers and family members becoming infected and enduring sickness and sometimes death.

> "I worked really hard to pull together some fabulous new
> data on MRSA to take back to one of the participating PD

units for an upcoming meeting. So the meeting comes and I said to the nurses: 'Guys, it's great news! Our work in improving hand hygiene and contact precautions is really paying off. Look, we went this long without an infection and that means we saved xxx hospital days because of lower length of stay and the lowered number of patients having to stay or die in the hospital.' And they just looked at me. They smiled and nodded but I could see they weren't really that excited. So I said: No, guys, this is really great news. Your work is paying off. See?'

"After a silence, with tears in her eyes, one of the nurses said, 'So, you mean that because of our work six people went home to their families and lives and jobs who would've died otherwise?'

"The nurse in this case knew exactly what mattered to her and found a way to translate the infection control data about length of stay, costs, hand hygiene and compliance into what mattered most to her."

David Hares, MD, MBA, Albert Einstein Medical Center,
In-house Facilitator

"Performance data seemed powerful and motivating when it provided a link between behavior and outcomes (for example, tracking and announcing the number of days without a transmission of MRSA) and helped foster a real sense of ownership and action."

Sharon Benjamin, PhD, PD Coach

Inventing Ways to Measure Impact

Each of the Beta Sites developed interesting "proxy" measures for assessing how well PD was working. In some sites these included indices such as the number of gown and gloves or soap and hand gel used hospital wide. In other places staff tracked the number of Discovery and Action Dialogues or the number of staff that participated in improvs. In every case where PD processes ignited real change, we saw proxy measures on performance being kept by participating staff. Often these measures were supported by feedback from the quality or infection control team but the ownership of the data was clearly fixed at the unit level. It appeared as the project unfolded that those hospitals where the units had the most ownership of data were also the units that had the best performance on reducing MRSA infections.

> "The nurse who decided to find out how many gowns they were using… I remember her saying. 'If I can count my son's underwear to find out if he is changing, we can do this'."
>
> *Jon Lloyd, MD, PD Coach*

More Invitations, More Answers

The hospitals engaged in Positive Deviance all had experience with participatory management and some had demonstrated excellence in this area. As a result, it was initially difficult for the hospital teams to believe that a much more robust engagement of staff was possible or needed. Yet one of the essential elements of the PD approach involves dramatically expanding the solution space by engaging "unusual suspects"—the people whose opinions have not traditionally been sought. If infection control initiatives are focused only on doctors and nurses, the good ideas of all the other individuals who contribute to patient care are lost.

Widely dispersed individuals in the hospital community itself become the thinkers and actors responsible for the success of the PD "solutions" and, equally important, the driving force behind the many iterations of discovery and action that characterize the PD approach.

> "The last group I worked with was the physicians; on other causes I would be talking to physicians first. Here you talk

to people on the front lines. It is more relevant to them. In the hospital, the physician sees a patient for a few minutes a day. They are never going to be impacted like the daily workers who do most of the patient care. The physicians are not as involved."

Wendy Ziai,MD,
Assistant Professor of Neurology, Neurosurgery, and Anesthesiology and Critical Care Medicine, The Johns Hopkins Hospital,
In-house Facilitator

"Getting environmental services staff to talk was easier than we expected. When we closed the door, they would talk. When our PD Coach Mark Munger was visiting, we asked if he might meet with neurology and neurosurgery. We asked for five minutes on the agenda; it turned into a whole hour. It turned out to be a pretty great conversation."

Linda Goss, ARNP,
Director, Infection Control and Vascular Access Nurses,
University of Louisville Hospital,
In-house Facilitator

The practice of Positive Deviance also means an ongoing effort to expand the conversation, make it more inclusive. "Unlikely suspects" are sought out for their perspectives and ideas. The phrase "nothing about me without me" reminds the group that their discussion needs to include anyone who is concerned with the issue. It is common practice at the end of a DAD to identify who else needs to be invited to the next meeting to discuss the issue more fully.

"Unlikely suspects" were responsible for many innovations at the Beta Site hospitals. There were established protocols for hand hygiene and isolation precautions, but none for the transport of infected patients through the hospital for tests or treatment. So transporters worked with caregivers and infection control professionals to develop the needed procedures, often playing out common scenes to discover where the risks were. A team from

Environmental Services at VA Pittsburgh developed checklists for cleaning rooms, identifying daily tasks and extra cleaning to be done after a patient was discharged. Jon Lloyd commented, "Proper room cleaning is as important for infection control as inserting a central line—and we do it far more often."

Hospital chaplains began using plastic covers on their Bibles so they could be cleaned with disinfectant wipes between patient visits. Physical therapists in long-term care units worked with infection control to develop safe procedures for taking patients out of their rooms for walks and physical therapy. All these diverse efforts solved specific challenges, and also helped to create collective mindfulness about the daily opportunities for transmission of infection.

Changing the Change Agents

Becoming Invisible

PD Coach Lisa Kimball, PhD, recalls getting a phone call from one of the managers at a PD hospital late in the day. The manager was driving home and said to Lisa "Well, the project's going pretty well but it's unnerving. If the staff on the units are doing the work, I keep wondering what I'm supposed to be doing."

In the sites where PD truly ignited, there were moments when the managers who, having unleashed the creativity and problem-solving of the staff, had to stand back and shift their thinking about their own roles. Mid and senior level managers had to shift from being the experts with answers to being facilitators who supported others. This shift, one of the most profound and elusive in PD, left many PD coaches and in-house facilitators feeling unmoored. As the project went along, they learned again and again the power of asking new questions fueled by a newly acquired and genuine curiosity.

In-house facilitators also struggled with the seductive allure of sliding back into the "expert" role. This was encouraged by staff who often expected to be "told" what to do. David Hares recalls being told by a group of nurses on one of the AEMC units: "We don't need to discuss this, just tell us what to do, sir, and we'll do it. Yes, sir!" Yet, the key concept of Positive Deviance is that the discovery process must be done by the persons whose behavior needs to change.

"The power—when we actually do it—of turning the whole discovery process over to the people whose behavior needs to change is intense. I've been working with organizational change for 30 years. Truly handing the discovery process to the front line people is rare, but it happens in PD."

Joelle Everett, MS, PD Coach

With time and continued practice, new roles and behavior came more naturally.

"There's a neat term—lineament—and it's the residue that repetitive practice leaves on the virtuoso. Violinists always have that callous under the chin where the violin rubs. Right-handed tennis players have hypertrophied arms on their serving side. So there is a physical imprint that repetitive practice leaves, so there are developed skills from persistence, and they can also be behavioral."

Jon Lloyd, MD, PD Coach

The Bridge to Culture Change is Ready for Passage

The coaches, most with long experience working with organizational change, were surprised to discover that in focusing on a rather narrow objective they were seeing significant behavioral and cultural change in the hospitals. Unlike some projects where changing the culture is an objective, the purpose of this project was to eliminate MRSA infections. Yet because PD practices foster powerful ownership and widespread staff engagement, the culture in the hospitals also changed.

One of the solutions that emerged from a Discovery and Action Dialogue at Hospital Pablo Tobon Uribe was having the guards suggest hand hygiene compliance for everyone entering and leaving the ward. But one day, one of those "everyones" was the hospital director general. The security guard had to remind him to wash his hands and to his credit he complied, thanked the guard, and told the story around the hospital. This story, as you can imagine, is regularly re-told.

When patient safety becomes the first concern, when volunteers step forward and find their ideas are heard and taken seriously, the results go far beyond the decrease in infections.

Beta Site leaders were gathered in Philadelphia for a conference at the close of the grant project. During a debrief activity at the close of the meeting, PD MRSA Prevention Partnerships CDC member John Jernigan turned to Jennifer Leachman, DPT, physical therapist at Billings Clinic and an enthusiastic member of the Billings Players and said, "I know that Billings is rechecking their infection rates, to make sure they are not accidentally overstated. What if the numbers are not so good?"

"So what?" Jennifer replied. "I know what PD has done for the hospital, and I know what it has done for me. I don't care about the numbers!"

Change is Here to Stay: Smile When Someone Calls You a Deviant

Two years after the end of the PD MRSA grant project, the influence of Positive Deviance continues. At some sites, there are still identified PD initiatives and new problems like diabetes management and end-of-life care that are being tackled. At others, PD is no longer a defined initiative, but part of "how we do things here." While the impact of PD has been measured, and demonstrated positive results reducing MRSA rates, the path and trajectory of spread is not readily quantified using standard methods.

Following the initial kick-off, which was open to all hospital staff, the priorities, actions and sequence of engagement of units was based on interest and self-selection. The social proof (demonstration that MRSA transmissions can be reduced within the hospital) becomes the catalyst that draws in new units. Because each engaged unit has a wide spectrum and large number of activated staff members, additional spread is often triggered through the relationships among staff members. Capitalizing on these strong, often invisible social networks is a special feature of PD and underlies its pattern of exponential growth within communities. Social network maps created by the Billings Clinic and VAPHS demonstrate these pathways for spread. For in-house facilitators, following the energy and interest of staff reduced the need to divert resources to overcome indifference among units not ready or interested in intervention.

In health care, sustained change is exceedingly rare. In PD sustained change is the norm, and ironically is greatest when the intervention itself seems to have disappeared. As staff ownership becomes more complete the PD intervention and involvement of in- house facilitators becomes less evident. The previously deviant behaviors become the new norm. Frequently, the behavior change skills learned during the PD intervention become unconsciously routine among in-house facilitators and the peers they influence.

"Something has changed, so complex nobody can put their finger on it. PD does something to people in the organization. Smile when you call people a deviant. I can't say what we've learned. We've learned a lot. There was never a point when we became different. When someone sees a problem and fixes it without telling you that is different. People can do that and not even think about it."

Patricia Norstrand MS, RN BC,
Senior Director, Department of Quality, Risk and Safety,
Franklin Square Hospital Center, In-house Facilitator

"*Have you changed?* I've definitely changed my behavior, yes. It's been unconscious over time. I have changed the way I approach other problems. It's a well-defined approach: how do you pose a question, listen for answers, get information from different people, delegate to different people? We now have 'huddles' in ICU units—all staff, five minutes, go over the daily plan. We talk about hygiene, and speaking up. It's a good way to start the day and share information."

Wendy Ziai, MD, Assistant Professor of Neurology, Neuro-
surgery, and Anesthesiology and Critical Care Medicine,
The Johns Hopkins Hospital, In-house Facilitator

"At Billings Clinic we are still using improv to explore complex situations. Recently, while playing out an improv scene, the operating room staff discovered that no one was wiping down (with disinfectant) some pieces of equipment. They explored when gloves should be removed and hands rewashed during surgery, such as after intubating a patient. Some complained that there was not time for repeated hand washing. But one physician spoke up, quietly and firmly, 'We have the time'."

Nancy Iversen, RN, CIC, Director of Patient Safety and Infection
Control, Billings Clinic, In-house Facilitator

"At the University of Louisville what has stuck is staff involvement. We are finding and interacting with people we haven't normally interacted with for infection control," said Linda Goss. "When we have a meeting," added Deanna Parker, "what is on the forefront of our minds is 'Who should be there?' Not just the managers."

Linda Goss, ARNP, Director,
Infection Control and Vascular Access Nurses,
Deanna Parker, BSN, Clinical Manager,
Medical Intensive Care Unit,
University of Louisville Hospital, In-house Facilitator

Post Script

While the grant and formal project work outlined here has ended, the story, like all good organizational stories, has not.

We hope it is evident from the material presented here that PD—though sometimes elusive—can be both powerful and effective.

And, as we conclude, we realized that like all heroic journeys we've returned to our starting place transformed—from expert to seeker; from teacher to explorer; from being resigned to HAIs to knowing they can be eliminated. Our world view, our vocabulary and our understanding of how things are possible all changed.

These changes, rooted in practice, are subtle, profound and often invisible. And, they open a wide gap between those with the experience and those who haven't traveled this road. Like mastery of all types we find ourselves wondering "how the world could have been otherwise?"

If good teaching is based on being able to remember what it is like not to know something, the challenge in coming back to share what we've learned about PD is to remember how we approached problem solving before PD.

A small story, then, to close. When asked how she knew the PD work had been successful, Maureen Jordon, head of respiratory and central supply at AEMC had lots of good evidence: changing practice in her unit with regard to HAIs; changing relationships with other staff in the hospital; improved respect and accountability. But she said the way she really knew the work had been successful was because her staff had changed how they worked so that PD practices had become the new norm.

We ourselves have been changed.

The journey is not over and we invite you to join us.

They have always had to extract every possible bit of goodness and nutrition from every scrap of land and fuel, economizing everywhere except with human labor and ingenuity, of which there is a surfeit.

— Nicole Mones, The Last Chinese Chef

Afterwords

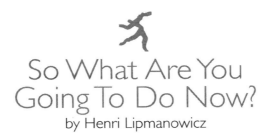

So What Are You Going To Do Now?

by Henri Lipmanowicz

If you are reading these lines it means you were interested enough to make it to the end of this book, unless of course you are someone who likes reading books from the end, in which case welcome and read on! The question for you now is what are you going to do with all these ideas?

With its multitude of data and stories, the description of such a big initiative as the PD MRSA Prevention Partnership can be overwhelming. At the risk of oversimplifying, let me boil down what was done and what made the difference into just one sentence, but one in which every word matters:

- **Invite everybody** affected to join others in discovering and or developing together more effective practices.

In contrast, the traditional approach to problem solving is:

- **Appoint a few people** to develop or import more effective practices and then try to impose them on everybody else.

The major objection we always hear to the approach we advocate is that including everybody is not practical—that it involves too many people, is too time-consuming, and is too chaotic and unwieldy. Unfortunately, in practice there is no choice. Indeed all who are affected will eventually have to be included, at the latest during the implementation of new practices. At that time the all-elusive "buy-in" will have to be actively sought. Lots of presentations will be made to "sell" the new ideas, and education and training campaigns will be deployed to try and bring along all the people who were left out during the development and decision phase. In large organizations this process takes weeks, months or years and, even with a big investment of time and resources, often fails to achieve desired results simply because in the end, people don't buy in. Excluding people from developing solutions to complex issues for which they are responsible makes them feel ignored, manipulated, threatened, and unappreciated. That leads to unenthusiastic and ineffective implementation, or worse.

Just remember how you feel when you are treated like this...

Leaders and managers are diminished by these buy-in tactics, and often caught in the middle between what comes down from the top and resistance from below. Rather than pushing, we have assembled a variety of effective approaches for including people and inviting them to take more responsibility. We call them Liberating Structures.[1]

So the choice is not whether to include or not include everybody but when and how to do it: early during the development phase; later during the implementation; or a mix of both. This book contains many stories about the benefits of early inclusion when groups can self-discover their own solutions. Time invested during the development phase is more than made up later by rapid and effective implementation by the people who already understand the plans and believe in them because they contain the solutions they developed with their community.

However, how to include people remains a challenge, particularly in organizations where there is no tradition for doing so. It is likely that even those who are enthusiastic about such an idea never had opportunities to learn inclusive methods. A variety of these Liberating Structures were used by participating hospitals, and this book described in detail two that were used extensively and proved their effectiveness:

- Discovery and Action Dialogue (DAD)

- Improv

Since you chose to read this book, I am quite sure that both can be of value to you. But there is only one sure way to find out...experiment at a scale that is comfortable for you. You don't need to wait for a huge problem like MRSA, or to work in health care, to discover the value of a DAD or an Improv. Both can be used routinely for engaging groups around much smaller problems. Find someone to partner with who likes the idea and, together, try out each method a few times.

The biggest hurdle always is getting over the angst of letting go of control. We will not know until the end what will come out of the group conversations or improvisations, and anyone using an unfamiliar method faces the unsettling question: "Am I going to make a fool of myself?" Fortunately both methods are resilient and forgiving; there is no need to be an expert at facilitation to generate useful outcomes. The simple fact of fully engaging a group of people and liberating their energy and creativity will yield valuable insights, certainly more so than a traditional meeting could.

Confidence builds with practice as it becomes gradually easier to *trust the people and trust the process* and to remain calm when the unavoidable messiness emerges. Traditional approaches hide their messiness behind the closed-door meetings of task forces and exclude any mention of it during presentations. Open-ended processes, however, make the indispensable messiness associated with discovery and development visible to all participants: **no mess = no innovation**! In a culture that conditions us to believe that **messy = bad management** that does take some getting used to.

If your interest in this book stems from a desire to try our approach for addressing a complex problem that affects a large number of people, I wouldn't recommend that you embark on such an ambitious project alone. Coaching support to help you get started is indispensable. In this case contacting one of the organizations that have experienced the whole MRSA process could be a useful starting point. Even if your initiative has nothing to do with MRSA or health care, people who have experienced success with open-ended processes can discuss your questions and share ideas on possible new directions for tackling your issues. A vibrant and supportive community of practice has emerged from the PD MRSA initiative; it is very welcoming to new members. Plexus Institute can help you find connections or locate a helping hand.

Thousands of lives and billions of dollars are waiting to be saved by reducing MRSA infections. Huge benefits are also waiting to be discovered in other domains both inside and outside of health care. Finally, at the personal level, learning how to be an inclusive leader is a transformative experience that opens the door to many new possibilities.

Thank you for joining this journey,

Henri Lipmanowicz

Henri Lipmanowicz is chair of the Plexus Institute Board of Trustees. He retired after a distinguished career at Merck, where he was president of the Merck Intercontinental and Japan Division, and a member of the Management Committee.

1. H. Lipmanowicz, and K. McCandless, "Liberating structures: innovating by including and unleashing everyone," *Performance*, vol. 2, no. 3, 2010, 6-20 http://www.ey.com/Publication/vwLUAssets/Liberating_structures/$FILE/Liberating%20structures.pdf (accessed 6-29-10)

Engagement, Affirmation, and Emergence
by Anthony L. Suchman

There is so much to learn from this book! It contains a wealth of principles and practices, and inspiring stories from around the world. From my perspective as a student and practitioner of organizational change, there are three themes I'd like to highlight that have important practical implications for change agentry.

The first and most important theme, *engaging and empowering all the people who are involved in the change*, has been richly described throughout the book. I can think of only one small point to add. I sometimes wonder if Positive Deviance is really the right name for this method. It puts primary emphasis on the people in every group who have developed innovative solutions. While there's no doubt that they are a valuable resource, what's most remarkable to me about PD is the way it intentionally takes traditional assumptions about where the expertise and decision-making are or should be located and turns them on their head. The outside consultants stay in the background, supporting the internal change leaders and encouraging them to keep themselves in the background so that the volunteers and the "unusual suspects" can take up their own authority and leadership. This resonates with what Peter Block wrote about power in his book *Stewardship*, one of the early manifestos for empowerment:

> Stewardship can be most simply defined as giving order to the dispersion of power. It requires us to systematically move choice and resources closer and closer to the bottom and edges of the organization. Leadership, in contrast, gives order to the centralization of power.[1]

You couldn't ask for a better illustration of the dispersion of power than the stories in the preceding pages. So maybe we could call the method "power dispersion" or "an organizational headstand" or something...

A second theme is that of *trying to fix what's wrong by looking for what's right*. What a wonderful paradox that is! We are seldom mindful of the way we cast out our attention, yet it is absolutely fateful. How we focus our attention, for instance whether we seek deficiencies or capacities, determines what we perceive. What we perceive becomes the basis for the interpretations and assumptions we make—the stories we tell ourselves about a given situation or organization or person. The stories become the basis of our expectations for the future, which then shape our actions and the reactions that we get. Our expectations also focus our attention and filter our subsequent perceptions. If you are starting to get the idea that this is all terribly self-fulfilling, you are completely right. This was the point of those legendary experiments about labeling rats maze-bright or maze-dull or children as having high or low IQs (when in fact there were no differences) and having the groups' performance shift in the direction of the artificially induced expectation. So let's be more mindful and intentional about how we cast out our attention.

Positive Deviance and its close cousin Appreciative Inquiry[2] are approaches that focus attention on what's right and how we can do more of it rather than what's wrong and how to do it less. They both are highly relational and make extensive use of stories as well. The curious thing is that the behaviors that come to light are often the exact same behaviors that would be discussed in the more traditional problem solving (what's wrong) approach, but with an opposite emotional spin (competence versus deficiency). And that emotional spin makes all the difference with regard to people adopting change or fighting it. The stories in this book illustrate people becoming excited, proud and motivated as they experience their own creativity and effectiveness. Who responds that way to being told what to do, or hearing that they are somehow deficient, that they are the problem? Looking for problems (the "pathologizing gaze") is a long-standing habit in both clinical and management professions. It's what we were all taught to do; there never were any alternatives. Now there are, and they work better. Let's use them.

The third theme I'd point to is that of *emergent design*. Given current prevailing images of leadership, it would take a lot of courage for a leader to say, "We have a clear goal—we need to eliminate hospital-acquired MRSA infections. I'm not sure how we'll get there, but I'd like to have you join with me to figure out the first step. And once we've taken that step, we'll have a better idea of the second step, and then the third one, and so on. We'll need to make this up as we go along, and we'll get there." This is how organizational change really happens in our nonlinear, self-organizing world.[3] Why is it so hard to tell the truth about this? Somehow our collective thinking has been hijacked by unrealistic expectations of control that are actually harmful, and we feel considerable pressure to keep up the pretense for fear of not looking like good and wise leaders. But as we've seen throughout this book, a really good leader is willing to "not know" and to engage as many people as possible in finding the path and figuring out the answers together.

Engagement, affirmation and emergence: powerful principles that offer practical guidance in the moment to moment work of organizational change. Gratitude and congratulations to the authors and all the people whose work they describe for such fine demonstrations of these principles in action and for giving us hope that positive change is very possible.

Anthony L. Suchman, MD, MA

Anthony Suchman is a practicing internist, a clinical professor of medicine at the University of Rochester, and senior consultant in the Healthcare Consultancy of McArdle Ramerman & Co. Through his teaching and writing he is known as a leading proponent of a partnership-based clinical approach known as Relationship-centered Care, and is bringing these principles and practices into the realm of administration and organizational behavior.

1. P. Block, *Stewardship*, (San Francisco: Berrett-Kohler, 1993), 18.

2. J.M. Watkins, and B.J Mohr, *Appreciative Inquiry: Change at the Speed of Imagination*, (San Francisco: Jossey-Bass/Pfeiffer, 2001).

3.   A.L. Suchman, "Organizations as machines, organizations as conversations: two core metaphors and their consequences," (*Medical Care* 2010: in press).

Networks, Possibilities, and Change
by Ori Brafman

This book tells some powerful stories of the role of social networks in driving innovation. The hospitals that teamed up with Plexus Institute and the Positive Deviance Initiative created networks of people from every part of their organizations. A new capacity for everyone to contribute solutions to some very serious problems in health care emerged with the growth of new relationships and collaborations.

In our research on how distributed social networks are affecting the nonprofit, government and business worlds, we discovered an intriguing analogy from the world of biology. Think about two species: spiders and starfish.[1]

A spider has a tiny head and eight legs coming out of a central body. While it can survive after losing a leg—maybe even two—it can't survive without its head.

A starfish doesn't have a head. Its central body isn't even in charge. In fact, the major organs are replicated throughout each and every arm. A starfish is a network of cells without the central control of a brain. If you cut off a spider's head it dies, but if you cut off a starfish's leg, it grows a new one, and that leg can grow into an entirely new starfish.

Organizations can be understood as being more or less like spiders or starfish. It turns out there are many competitive advantages for organizations that operate more like starfish, as illustrated by the success of entities like Craigslist and Alcoholics Anonymous, which demonstrate power-ful flexibility and resilience. The extraordinary results achieved by the proj-ects described in this book illustrate how the ideas and conditions that create successful and sustained organizational innovation also apply to change initiatives.

A centralized organization or initiative is easy to understand. You have a clear leader who is in charge, and there's a specific place where decisions are made. Planning is aimed at being efficient and consistent in how rules are made, disseminated and implemented. These traditional "spiders" have a rigid hierarchy and top down leadership. Change initiatives tend to be mandated from the top and implemented with organization-wide roll-outs, standardized training, a small group of managers assigned to lead the change, and a calendar of pre-planned activities. The problem is how man-dated change can be sustained after the initial fanfare. When leadership at the top changes, the initiative is often left to wither on the vine while some new effort is launched. Staff turnover results in lost knowledge and, with-out significant new investment in training, momentum stalls.

In contrast, the stories in this volume speak to efforts that have been sustained over time and continue to thrive and grow long after the initial introduction. These initiatives rely on the power of peer relationships and embody a number of key principles that create conditions for significant change.

The Power of Chaos: While the traditional roll-out of change initia-tives is based on developing and distributing a standardized message and method, the PD approach developed by the participating hospitals with Plexus Institute and the Positive Deviance Initiative supports an emergent model that leverages the creative variance in a distributed network of ac-tivity. Starfish systems are incubators for creative, destructive, innovative or seemingly crazy ideas because they don't start with a set of pre-deter-mined solutions. Instead, new ideas can bubble up, sometimes from sur-prising places, and attract attention and adoption by people who can pick them up and run with them on their own initiative. Positive Deviance is a process for uncovering and experimenting with new ideas that just might work even if they come from "unusual suspects."

Knowledge at the Edge: For change to really take hold, knowledge must be spread throughout the organization. A recurring theme in the stories in this volume about hospitals is that expertise and knowledge that was previously the purview of infection control departments and medical professionals evolved into being much more widely shared. MRSA is sometimes described as a "toucher's" problem, meaning that anyone who touches anyone or anything in a hospital can play a role in transmission. That implies that whether you are greeting visitors or performing surgery, you can make a significant difference in stopping MRSA transmission, and thus your knowledge about how your behavior impacts the problem is critical to the solution.

Everyone Wants to Contribute: People in innovative organizations not only have knowledge but want to share that knowledge and use it to make a difference. This book is full of examples of how inviting *everyone* to participate creates an environment of peer-to-peer support and the discovery of new ways to get around obstacles to implementing desired behaviors. The PD mantra "go and ask them" speaks to the power of going directly to the people on the front lines to find out how they see the problem and listen to their ideas about how to solve it.

Catalysts Rule: Starfish organizations rely on catalysts rather than traditional leaders. A catalyst gets a decentralized organization going and then gets out of the way so that its members can take charge going forward. That doesn't mean that those in the organization with "position power" have no role. Particularly in organizations (like hospitals) with a strong tradition of hierarchy, leaders need to send the right signals about how the initiative will be supported and the extent to which there is an openness to ideas and efforts that come from the bottom up. But the stories in this book are about the power of facilitative leadership to catalyze activities and encourage new leaders to step forward and make things happen in their own domains.

Measure, Monitor and Manage: It would be a misconception to think that just because grassroots driven initiatives tend to be ambiguous and unpredictable, their results are not possible to track and measure. However, there are some key differences from the typical approach we use to assess a change initiative. Traditional approaches ask questions like: How soon will everyone attend the roll out presentation? How many people have been trained? How well are units adhering to the plan? As we see in the examples included here, the interest is more in the health of the network where new questions become important: Do members continue participating? Is the network growing? Is it spreading? Is it mutating? Are new leaders emerging? Ironically, one of the best indicators this more people-driven initiative is becoming successful is the extent to which things are happening that initial organizers didn't have a hand in creating and maybe don't even know anything about!

The most important thing to remember is that at first glance, starfish movement can appear disorganized and lacking a concrete focus. But appearances can be misleading. In many cases, whether Alcoholics Anonymous, the women's suffrage movement in the United States, the peer-to-peer music sharing sites, or teams of people trying to solve critical problems in health care, these networks can change the world. They're effective, in fact, because they lack hierarchical structure, and therefore can adapt and innovate in ways that spiders cannot.

Ori Brafman

Ori Brafman has been a life-long entrepreneur in business, government, and the nonprofit sector. He is the author of best-selling books including: The Starfish and the Spider: The Unstoppable Power of Leaderless Organizations; Sway: The Irresistible Pull of Irrational Behavior; and Click: The Magic of Instant Connections.

1.   O. Brafman and R. Beckstrom, *The Starfish and the Spider: The Unstoppable Power of Leaderless Organizations,* (New York: Penguin Group USA, 2006).

Innovative, Ancient, and Powerful
by Jeffrey Goldstein

From my perspective as a theorist and practitioner of complexity science applied to organizations, I was pleasantly startled when I first heard Jerry Sternin speak about PD. Curt and Henri had invited me to accompany them to a symposium where Jerry was one of the speakers. It only took a couple of minutes into his presentation before I was struck by how profound PD was in solving long-standing social problems. What Jerry was saying about PD had a strange affect on me. On the one hand, it seemed to be such an incredibly innovative and powerful social and organizational intervention. On the other hand, there was something about PD that struck me as ancient in the way it spoke of what already was present in communities, had always been present, and only needed skillful means to be actualized.

To be sure, there was also the extraordinary manner in which Jerry was communicating to the audience. This little guy was so much *larger than life:* his humanity, his brilliance, and most especially, the hope expressed in how PD could improve even situations previously thought intractable. Please note, Jerry was not the kind of speaker who drew attention to himself or some special properties he possessed. Instead, it was all about PD and the what and how of bringing about positive change that was always in the forefront of Jerry's work. I also left the meeting with the sense that PD dovetailed with several complexity sciences concepts and I was eager to learn as much as I could by sitting at the feet of the master.

It was partly my perception of Jerry being "larger than life" that really slammed me when I heard he had passed away. It took me awhile to get over the initial shock and deep dismay. Sure, I mourned for myself and for his family and friends that we would no longer be able to sit at his feet, be uplifted by his truly inspiring stories and teachings, his good humor and ebullience, his way of seeing beyond petty concerns to what was truly important in any situation. I mourned also for the concern he must have felt about the fate of PD. But it wasn't PD *per se* that was the focus of Jerry's life work. Rather, it was the amelioration of whatever social or community need was being experienced wherever in the world he was called to work. PD was only one of the tools to achieve this, albeit one with great potency. It was this task of aiding humanity to a higher quality of life that really made Jerry larger than life. A glimpse of this quality can be found in the current book that explains the nuts and bolts of PD in improving lives all over the world, a book replete with wonderfully inspiring examples.

I also remember the many times when I participated with Jerry and his wife Monique in one of the first hospital interventions using Positive Deviance to decrease rates of MRSA and in other projects. It was both intellectually and might I say, *spiritually*, stimulating for me to have the opportunity of hanging around with the Sternins and observing how they transmitted the essentials of PD to different people in the hospital, as well as talking with Jerry and Monique about how I saw PD dovetailing with complexity science concepts and their social applications.

The intersection of PD and complexity science becomes evident, I believe, in an examination of how innovation comes about in complex systems. From a complexity science lens, one crucial way innovation happens is by small "seeds" or experiments in novelty that are then amplified to spread through the system. For certain reasons having to do with the dynamics of complex systems, fluctuations and perturbations are going on all the time but usually are negligible in their effect. It is like a calm-looking lake when there's no wind. The surface is like a mirror and it seems that nothing at all is going on beneath this placid surface. However, if a sensitive probe were to be placed in the lake, this probe would detect all sorts of small currents moving in many different directions because of the fish and turtles and frogs and water bugs swimming around in addition to other currents coming from underground springs. These small currents are "seeds" of difference that can become intensified and spread under the right conditions, or in Jerry's language, the positive deviances, that can function to shift a social system so that its members' lives are improved.

One of the really fantastic ideas of PD and complexity science is that these experiments in novelty, these departures from the norm, don't need to be created. They are already there! The promising ones have the potential to become powerful instruments of change throughout the system if they are noticed and disseminated. Jerry's genius was to recognize this phenomena in human social systems and then to find ways of disseminating the positive deviances through means of the system's *own* resources. And that meant there would be little chance for what Jerry called an "immune reaction"—the resistance that often arises when outside experts try to impose some kind of change.

I also remember the time when I was in Cork, Ireland at a conference where Jerry and I were two of the speakers. One early evening, Jerry and I were walking along one of the roads next to the campus of University College. Five students were approaching from the opposite direction. They appeared to be graduate students because of their age and bearing. And they were Chinese. What happened next I am sure is the first and last time it will happen in my life. Jerry said hello to them in their own language and then commenced to hold a full blown conversation with them! Their jaws dropped just as mine did. Here was an American man, in Ireland, talking to them fluently in their language! This story reveals not only Jerry's genius linguistic abilities, but I think even more important, how he was able to cross over barriers, cultural, social, and human, and to do so with *healing bridges*.

Jerry also knew the Chinese classics, the books of Chinese wisdom such as the great book of Taoism, the *daodejing*. He was an embodiment of how that book described leadership: the focus is not on the leader's personality or special charisma. On the contrary, it is a kind of leadership that vanishes in the work that is accomplished. This book is another crucial step in that much needed direction.

Jeffrey Goldstein, PhD

Jeffrey Goldstein, PhD, is full professor at the Adelphi University School of Business, Garden City, New York. He is the author or editor of numerous books including: Complexity and the Nexus of Leadership: Leveraging Nonlinear Science to Create Ecologies of Innovation; Complexity Science and Social Entrepreneurship: Adding Social Value through Systems Thinking; Complex Systems Leadership Theory; Annuals of Emergence: Complexity and Organization; Classic Complexity; and The Unshackled Organization.

Books and Articles Bibliography

- Anderson, R., Issel, L. and McDaniel, R. "Nursing homes as complex adaptive systems: relationship between management practice and resident outcomes," *Nursing Research,* vol. 52, no.1, 2003.

- Anderson, R., McDaniel, R., "Taking complexity science seriously: new research, new methods," in *On the Edge: Nursing in The Age of Complexity,* C. Lindberg, S. Nash, and C. Lindberg, eds., (Bordenown, NJ: PlexusPress, 2008).

- Blyth, R. H., *Haiku, Volume 1: Eastern Culture,* (Tokyo: Hokuseido, 1949).

- Chui, G., "Unified theory is getting closer, Hawking predicts," *San Jose Mercury News,* 2000, section A.

- Cohen, J., "Calming Traffic on Bogota's Killing Streets," *Science,* vol. 319, no. 5864, 2008.

- Committee on Quality of Health Care in America, Institute of Medicine, *Crossing the Quality Chasm, A New Health System for the 21st Century,* (Washington, D.C.: National Academy Press, 2001.)

- De Bary, W.T. and Bloom, I., *Sources of Chinese Tradition from the Earliest Times to 1600,* 2nd edition, (New York: Colombia University Press, 1999).

- De Bono, Edward *I am Right You are Wrong: From This to the New Renaissance: From Rock Logic to Water Logic,* 1st American edition, (New York: Viking Adult, 1992).

- Diamond, Jarred, *Guns, Germs and Steel: The Fates of Human Societies,* (New York/London: W.W. Norton & Co., 1999).

- Dorsey, D., "Positive Deviant," *Fast Company,* November 30, 2000.

- Giddens, Anthony, *The Constitution of Society: Outline of the Theory of Structuration,* (Berkeley: University of California Press, 1986).

- Glouberman, Sholom and Zimmerman, Brenda, "Complicated and complex systems: what would successful reform of medicine look like," in *Health Care Services and the Process of Change,* P. Forest, T. McKintosh and G. Marchilden, eds, (Toronto: University of Toronto Press, 2004).

- Goldberger, A., "Fractal variability versus pathologic periodicity: complexity loss and stereotypy in disease," *Perspectives in Biology and Medicine,* vol. 40, no. 4, 1997.

- Holland, John H., *Emergence: From Chaos to Order,* (Cambridge, MA: Perseus Books, 1998).

- Johnson, Steven, *The Ghost Map: The Story of London's Most Terrifying Epidemic—and How It Changed Science, Cities, and the Modern World,* (New York: Riverhead Books, 2006).

- Kauffman, Stuart, *At Home in the Universe: The Search for the Laws of Self-Organization and Complexity,* (New York: Oxford University Press, 1995).

- Kunreuther, Howard, and Useem, Michael, *Learning from Catastrophes: Strategies for Reaction and Response,* (Upper Saddle River, NJ: Wharton School Publishing, 2009).

- Lindberg, Claire, Nash, Sue and Lindberg, Curt, *On the Edge: Nursing in the Age of Complexity.* (Bordentown, NJ: PlexusPress, 2008).

- Lindberg, R. and Hutchens, D., "Edward O. Wilson Speaks on Complexity," *Emerging,* January/February, 2002.

- Lorenz, Edward N., *The Essence of Chaos,* (Seattle: University of Washington Press, 1993).

- Mackintosh, U. Marsh, D., and Schroeder, D., "Sustained positive deviant child care practices and their effects on child growth in Viet Nam," *Food and Nutrition Bulletin* 2002, vol.23, no. 4, (supplement).

- McDaniel, R. and Driebe, D., "Complexity science and health care management," in *Advances in Health Care Management,* vol. 2, J. Blair, M. Fottler, and G. Savage, eds., (Stamford, CT: JAI Press, 2001).

- McKenna, Maryn, *Superbug: The Fatal Menace of MRSA,* (New York City: Free Press, 2010).

- Miller, W., et al., "Practice jazz: understanding variation in family practice using complexity science," *The Journal of Family Practice,* vol. 50, no. 10, 2001.

- Morgan, Gareth, *Images of Organization,* updated edition, (Thousand Oaks: Sage Publications, Inc, 1997).

- Peterson, L.R., et al., "New Technology for Detecting Multi-resistant Pathogens in the Clinical Microbiology Laboratory," *Emerging Infections Disease,* vol. 7, no. 2, 306-311.

- Sachs, Jessica Snyder, *Good germs, bad germs: health and survival in bacterial world,* (New York: Hill and Wang, 2008).

- Scott, Douglas R., "The Direct Medical Costs of Healthcare-Associated Infections in U.S. Hospitals and the Benefits of Prevention," (Washington, D.C.: CDC, 2009).

- Sepkowitz, K., "Forever unprepared—the predictable unpredictability of pathogens," *The New England Journal of Medicine,* vol. 361, no. 2, 2009.

- Shafique, Muhammad, Sternin, Monique, and Singhal, Arvind, "Will Rahima's Firstborn Survive Overwhelming Odds? Positive Deviance for Maternal and Newborn Care in Pakistan," *Positive Deviance Wisdom Series, Number 5,* Boston, Tufts University: Positive Deviance Initiative, 2010.

- Singhal, Arvind and Dura, Lucia, *Protecting Children from Exploitation and Trafficking: Using the Positive Deviance Approach in Uganda and Indonesia,* (Save the Children, 2009).

- Singhal, A. and Greiner, K. G, "Performance activism and civic engagement through symbolic and playful actions," *Journal of Development Communication,* vol. 9, no. 2, 2008.

- Snow, John, *On the Mode of Communication of Cholera,* 2nd edition, (London: John Churchill, 1855).

- Sokoloff, Nancy B., *Three Victorian Women Who Changed Their World,* (London: Macmillan, 1982).

- Spellberg, Brad, *Rising Plague: The Global Threat from Deadly Bacteria and Our Dwindling Arsenal to Fight Them,* (Amherst, NY: Prometheus Books, 2009).

- Stacey, Ralph, *Complexity and Creativity in Organizations,* (San Francisco: Berrett-Kohler, Publishers, 1996).

- Stacey, Ralph, *Strategic Management and Organisational Dynamics: The Challenge of Complexity to Ways of Thinking About Organisations,* 5th edition, (London: Pearson Education, 2007).

- Strogatz, Steven, *Sync: The Emerging Science of Spontaneous Order,* (New York: Hyperion Books, 2003).

- West, Bruce, "A physicist looks at physiology," in *On the Edge: Nursing in the Age of Complexity,* C. Lindberg, S. Nash, and C. Lindberg, eds., (Bordentown, NJ: PlexusPress, 2008).

- West, Bruce, *Where Medicine Went Wrong: Rediscovering the Path to Complexity,* (Singapore: World Scientific, 2006).

- Westley, Francis, Zimmerman, Brenda, and Patton, Michael, *Getting to Maybe: How the World is Changed,* (Toronto: Random House Canada, 2006).

- Woodham-Smith, Cecil, *Florence Nightingale 1820 – 1910,* (London: Penguin, 1955).

- Zeitlin, M. Ghassemi, H, and Mansour, M., *Positive Deviance in Child Nutrition,* (New York: UN University Press, 1990).

- Zimmerman, Brenda, Plsek, Paul, and Lindberg, Curt, *Edgeware: Insights from Complexity Science for Health Care Leaders,* (Irving, TX: VHA, Inc., 1998).

Web Site Bibliography

- AbsoluteAstronomy.com, Florence Nightingale: Facts, Discussion Forum. http://www.absoluteastronomy.com/topics/Florence_Nightingale (accessed 6-17-10).

- Agency for Healthcare Research Quality (AHRQ), "AHRQ: 2009 National Healthcare Quality Report." http://www.ahrq.gov/qual/nhqr09/Key.htm (accessed 6-8-10).

- ARS Research, "Timeline-Story on Penicillin Research." http://www.ars.usda.gov/is/timeline/penicillin.htm (accessed 11-9-09).

- Bassler, Bonnie, "HHMI Scientist Bio: Bonnie L. Bassler, PhD," Howard Hughes Medical Institute, Biomedical Research & Science Education. http://www.hhmi.org/research/investigators/bassler_bio.html (accessed 6-7-10).

- BBC News, Millennial Bridge, "Watch the Bridge Wobble." http://news.bbc.co.uk/hi/english/static/in_depth/uk/2000/millennium_bridge/default.stm (accessed 6-4-10).

- Brock, Thomas, University of Wisconsin, "Brave New Biosphere," University of Wisconsin-Madison, 1999. http://whyfiles.org/022critters/hot_bact.html (accessed 3-30-10).

- Caballero, M. C., "Academic Turns City into a Social Experiment: Mayor Mockus of Bogotá and his Spectacularly Applied Theory." *Harvard Gazette*, November 2004. http://www.news.harvard.edu/gazette/2004/03.11/01-mockus.html (accessed 6-28-10).

- CDC, "Fact Sheet: Invasive MRSA, CDC Infection Control in Healthcare." Centers for Disease Control and Prevention. http://www.cdc.gov/ncidod/dhqp/ar_mrsa_Invasive_FS.html (accessed 12-24-09).

- CDC, "Overview: HA-MRSA, CDC Infection Control in Healthcare." Centers for Disease Control and Prevention. http://www.cdc.gov/ncidod/dhqp/ar_mrsa.html (accessed 4-17-10).

• CDC, "Healthcare-Associated *Staphylococus aureus*, Overview of Health-care Associated MRSA," Centers for Disease Control and Prevention. http://www.cdc.gov/ncidod/dhqp/ar_mrsa.html (accessed 4-17-10).

• CDC, "Invasive MRSA," Centers for Disease Control and Prevention. http://www.cdc.gov/ncidod/dhqp/ar_mrsa_Invasive_FS.html (accessed 12-24-09).

• Cherry, Kendra, "Selected Quotations by Psychologist Kurt Lewin." http://psychology.about.com/od/psychologyquotes/a/lewinquotes.htm (accessed 6-23-10).

• Cohn, David, "Semmelweis," University of Louisville. "http://pyramid.spd.louisville.edu/~eri/fos/semmelweis.htmlSemmelweis (accessed 6-28-10).

• D'Elia, Tom, "In Hot Waters," The Why Files: The Science Behind the News. http://whyfiles.org/022critters/hot_bact.html (accessed 3-30-10).

• D'Elia, Tom, et al., "Isolation of Lake Vostok Accretion Ice," *Applied and Environmental Microbiology*, vol. 74, no. 15, August 2008, 4962-4965. http://www.ncbi.nlm.nih.gov/pmc/articles/PMC2519340/pdf/2501-07.pdf (accessed 3-15-10).

• Duke Medicine and Communications, "New Superbug Surpasses MRSA Infection Rates in Community Hospitals." http://www.dukehealth.org/health_library/news/new_superbug_surpasses_mrsa_infection_rates_in_community_hospitals (accessed 4-17-10).

• Ho, David, "TIME 100: Alexander Fleming," Time Inc. Portal. http://205.188.238.181/time/time100/scientist/profile/fleming.html (accessed 3-5-10).

• "Hospital-Acquired Infections, MRSA Killed 48,000 Americans In One Year." *Medical News Today*: Health News. http://www.medicalnewstoday.com/articles/180065.php (accessed 4-17-10).

• Lipmanowicz, H. and McCandless, K., "Liberating structures: innovating by including and unleashing everyone," *Performance*, vol. 2, no. 3, 6-20, http://www.ey.com/Publication/vwLUAssets/Liberating_structures/$FILE/Liberating%20structures.pdf (accessed 6-29-10).

• Loudon, Irvine, "Semmelweis and his thesis," National Center for Biotechnology Information. http://www.ncbi.nlm.nih.gov/pmc/articles/PMC1299347 (accessed 6-16-10).

- McNeil, Donald, "Fly Away Home." *The New York Times*, October 3, 2006. http://www.nytimes.com/2006/10/03/sci ence/03butter.html?_r=3&ref=science&oref=slo (accessed 6-23-10).

- *Medical News Today*, "Hospital Acquired Infections, MRSA killed 48,000 Americans in One Year," 3-23-10, report from February 22 *Archives of Internal Medicine*. http://www.medicalnewstoday.com/articles/180065.php (accessed 4-17-10).

- Mockus, A, *América Latina, Consensos y Paz Social*, Presentation at the 34th Congreso Internacional de Co-industria, Caracas, Venezuela, June 30, 2004. Retrieved from http://conindustria.org/CONGRESO2004/Intervenci%C3%B3n%20Antan as%20Mockus.pdf (accessed 6-29-10).

- Norwegian Refugee Council, Internally Displaced Peoples (IDPs) in Colombia, "New Displacement Continues, Response Still Ineffective," Internal Displacement Monitoring Centre. http://www.internal-displacement.org/countries/colombia (accessed 5-25-10).

- PoetsTree, ThePoetsTree.com, Odyssey Press, Inc. http://www.thepoetstree.com/index.php (accessed 6-29-10).

- Rockerfeller University, The Rockefeller University Newswire, "Researchers track evolution and spread of drug-resistant bacteria across hospitals and continents." http://newswire.rockefeller.edu/?page=engine&id=1024 (accessed 6-7-10).

- *Science Daily*, "Explaining Why The Millennium Bridge Wobbled," *Science Daily*: News & Articles in Science, Health, Environment & Technology. http://www.sciencedaily.com/releases/2005/11/051103080801.htm (accessed 6-10-10).

- *Science News*, "Math Trek," Florence Nightingale: Passionate Statistician. www.sciencenews.org/view/access/id/38939/title/jr_mtrek_nightingale (accessed 6-10-17).

- UCLA School of Public Health, "John Snow—a historical giant in epidemiology," UCLA School of Public Health. http://www.ph.ucla.edu/epi/snow.html (accessed 6-23-10).

- Urban, Laura, "Tough microbes to treat toxins?" *The Scientist, Magazine of Life Sciences*. http://www.the-scientist.com/blog/display/57342 (accessed 6-2-10).

- UCMP-University of California Museum of Paleontology, "Antony van Leeuwenhoek." http://www.ucmp.berkeley.edu/history/leeuwenhoek.html (accessed 5-5-10).

- USDA, "ARS Research Timeline-Story on Penicillin Research." http://www.ars.usda.gov/is/timeline/penicillin.htm (accessed 11-9-09).

- Waggoner, Ben, "Antony van Leeuwenhoek," UCMP - University of California Museum of Paleontology. http://www.ucmp.berkeley.edu/history/leeuwenhoek.html (accessed 5-10-10).

- Wikipedia, "Ignz Semmelweis." http//en.wikipedia.org/wiki/Ignaz_Semmelweis (accessed 5-10-10).

- Wikipedia, "John Snow (physician)." http://en.wikipedia.org/wiki/John_Snow_(physician) (accessed 6-23-10).

- Wikipedia, "Oliver Wendell Holmes, Sr." http://en.wikipedia.org/wiki/Oliver_Wendell_Holmes,_Sr (accessed 5-5-10).

- Wong, George, "Penicillin, The Wonder Drug," University of Hawaii at Manoa, Botany. http://www.botany.hawaii.edu/faculty/wong/BOT135/Lect21b.htm (accessed 11-15-09).

Acknowledgements

The editors would like to extend their deep appreciation to all who gave of their time, expertise and passion to make this book possible. First on our acknowledgement list must be the members of the PD MRSA Prevention Partnership who did something that had not been done before—employ Positive Deviance (PD) on a significant scale in health care to address a major public health challenge, the prevention of health care-associated infections. In many ways staff from the participating hospitals and their PD coaches wrote the story on which this book is based. The organizational members of the PD MRSA Prevention Partnership were: Albert Einstein Medical Center, Philadelphia, PA; Billings Clinic, Billings, MT; Franklin Square Hospital Center, Baltimore, MD; The Johns Hopkins Hospital, Baltimore, MD; University of Louisville Hospital, Louisville, KY; Veterans Administration Pittsburgh Healthcare System, Pittsburgh, PA; Hospital El Tunal, Bogota, Colombia; Hospital Pablo Tobon Uribe, Medellin, Colombia; Plexus Institute; Positive Deviance Initiative: Centers for Disease Control and Prevention (CDC); and Delmarva Foundation. Individuals who served as PD coaches for the hospitals were: Sharon Benjamin; Kevin Buck; Joelle Everett; Lisa Kimball; Henri Lipmanowicz; Jon Lloyd; Keith McCandless; Mark Munger; Jerry Sternin; Monique Sternin; and Margaret Toth. John Jernigan, from the CDC, generously offered his expertise on infection prevention, epidemiology, and comparative measurement, plus probing questions and encouragement. John

Stelling worked along side John Jernigan in the effort to capture the impact of this initiative on infection rates. June Holley and Chris Black brought their social network mapping skills to this initiative and the pages of this book.

The Pioneer Portfolio of The Robert Wood Johnson Foundation provided a grant that helped support this endeavor. To the Foundation and Senior Program Officer, Rosemary Gibson, we extend our deep gratitude.

Several people played important roles in pulling this volume together and helping us reach the finish line. Joelle Everett and Deborah Cooney offered their expert copy editing and proofreading skills. Douglas Sharp worked on references. David Hutchens created the cover and interior design for the book. Lisa Kimball provided important organizational support and encouragement. Carlos Urrea and David Hares helped with communicating with our Spanish speaking colleagues in Colombia and in translating their contributions.

About Plexus Institute
and Positive Deviance Initiative

Plexus Institute (*www.plexusinstitute.org*) is a non-profit organization formed in 2001 by a small group of people from diverse backgrounds who shared a vision of fostering the health of individuals, families, communities, organizations and the natural environment by helping people use concepts from the new science of complexity. In the years since, Plexus has created and supported a large and growing community devoted to this purpose. With its members, trustees and science advisors, the Institute has pioneered the introduction of complexity science principles and practices in health care, nursing, education, and business. This has enabled members of the Plexus community to effectively address complex challenges. The infection prevention work described in this volume is an example of what is possible through tapping advances in complexity science and using processes that foster engagement, creative conversations, and new connections within organizations and communities. These processes, known within Plexus as Liberating Structures, include Positive Deviance, Open Space, Conversation Café, Group Consultations, and many others.

Plexus works diligently to share its complexity resources on its website, through regular postings to its members, during Plexus conferences and through its publishing arm, PlexusPress. *Inviting Everyone: Healing Health*

Care through Positive Deviance joins *On the Edge: Nursing in the Age of Complexity* as the second publication of PlexusPress.

Positive Deviance Initiative (*www.positivedeviance.org*), an affiliate of Tufts University Friedman School of Nutrition Science and Policy, is a network organization dedicated to amplifying the use of the Positive Deviance (PD) approach to enable communities worldwide to solve seemingly intractable problems that require behavioral and social change. The Initiative was founded by Jerry and Monique Sternin. Visit the Positive Deviance Initiative web site and read the Wisdom Series to learn how PD initiatives have improved the lives of people who face malnutrition, high rates of maternal and infant mortality, the need for child protection, the aftermath of war and the impact of poverty. The Positive Deviance Initiative welcomes stories from individuals and organizations about experiences they have with Positive Deviance.

Index

About the Authors and Editors

About the Editors, who also contributed much of the content in this book

- *Arvind Singhal,* PhD, is the Samuel Shirley and Edna Holt Marston Endowed Professor and director of the Social Justice Initiative in the Department of Communication, University of Texas at El Paso. He is also William J. Clinton Distinguished Fellow at the Clinton School of Public Service, Little Rock, Arkansas. Singhal teaches and conducts research in diffusion of innovations, organizing for social change, and entertainment-education. He is co-author or editor of 10 books and monographs including *Protecting Children from Exploitation and Trafficking: Using the Positive Deviance Approach; Communication of Innovations; Organizing for Social Change;* and *Combating AIDS: Communication Strategies in Action.* He has authored more than 150 peer-reviewed essays and received numerous awards for excellence in scholarship.

- *Curt Lindberg,* DMan, is chief learning and science officer of Plexus Institute and a founder of the organization. He has played an important role in introducing complexity science concepts and Positive Deviance into health care thinking and organizational management and practice. Lindberg is the author of numerous articles on complexity and co-author of the book *Edgeware: Insights From Complexity Science for Health Care Leaders*, and co-editor of the book *On the Edge: Nursing in the Age of Complexity*. In 2008 he received a Doctor of Management degree from the University of Hertfordshire, where he studied under Professor Ralph Stacey.

- *Prucia Buscell* is a former newspaper reporter and freelance writer who is now communications director of Plexus Institute. In her role at Plexus she has written extensively about complexity science and the use of Positive Deviance in health care.

About the Authors

- *Karlo Roberto Reyes Barrera,* RN, is a hospital administration specialist at Hospital El Tunal. In this capacity he helped coordinate the hospital's Positive Deviance-informed infection prevention effort.

- *Sharon Benjamin,* PhD, a self-described *"prac-ademic,"* consults with multi-lateral, NGO and health care organizations. An adjunct at New York University, she teaches the leadership capstone course for MPA students. Her work supports leaders seeking to effect profound transformation—within themselves and their organizations—using pioneering methods. She has been a member of the governing boards of almost two-dozen nonprofit organizations including Plexus Institute, BlueVoice.org, American Oceans Campaign, Earthworks and the advisory board of Oceana.

- *Lucia Dura* is a PhD candidate in the Rhetoric and Writing Studies program, Department of English, at University of Texas at El Paso. Her concentration is in public administration, and her research interests are rhetoric for social change, technical and professional writing, and organizational communication. Her dissertation uses the case of post-conflict reintegration in Northern Uganda to explore the extent of rhetorical awareness and rhetorical strategy involved in Positive Deviance.

- *Narda Maria Olarte Escobar,* MD, is an epidemiology specialist with Hospital El Tunal. In addition to her medical degree she has a master's in infections and tropical health. She has 10 years of experience in epidemiology and health care infection prevention and control, and helped lead the PD MRSA prevention work at her hospital.

- *Joelle Lyons Everett* is founding partner of Sound Resources, an international consulting firm based in Washington. Her diverse clients are often struggling to respond to changing circumstances, or working to create transformational change. She worked with Plexus Institute on the PD MRSA initiative. Everett is author of *Strange and Wonderful Things*, a book of original poems.

- *Andrea Restrepo Gouzy,* MD, studied general medicine, pediatrics and infectious diseases at the University of Antioquia in Medellín, Colombia. She was a Fellow for six months at Dallas Children Hospital, affiliated with The University of Texas. She is a pediatric infectious disease specialist at Hospital Pablo Tobón Uribe in Medellín, and an active member of the hospital's Infection Prevention Committee, the group responsible for leading the Positive Deviance initiative and the hand hygiene program.

- *Karen Greiner,* PhD, is a post-doctoral scholar at the University of South Florida where she conducts research and teaches classes. She served as a Peace Corps volunteer in Cameroon and a Fulbright Fellow in Colombia. She earned an MA in International Education from New York University and a PhD in Health Communication from Ohio University.

- *Ismael Alberto Valderrama Marquez,* RN, is a cardiology and respiratory specialist at Hospital El Tunal. He has extensive experience in epidemiology and health care infection prevention and control, and played an active role in the hospital's Positive Deviance MRSA prevention initiative.

- *Keith McCandless,* founding partner of the Social Invention Group in Seattle, is a consultant with expertise in innovating by including and unleashing everyone. He has co-developed Liberating Structures, a set of 33 practices that make it easy for groups of people to be creative, adaptable, build on each other's ideas, and get better than expected results. He calls himself a structured improvisationalist.

- *Margaret Toth,* MD, graduated with honors from Yale University School of Medicine and trained in internal medicine at the University of California at San Francisco. She worked as a practicing physician at the Cleveland Clinic and the Metro Medical Center in Cleveland. She served as a physician executive for Ohio KePro and the Delmarva Foundation. Toth worked with Jerry and Monique Sternin coaching hospitals in Maryland in their application of Positive Deviance to fight infection, and introduced the concept of PD to a larger group of hospitals during her tenure with Delmarva.

- *Carlos A. Urrea,* MD, was born in Medellin, Colombia, studied at Universidad Nacional de Colombia, where he earned his medical degree in 2001. He was awarded a Masters in Public Health at Johns Hopkins University in 2008. He is currently the director of patient safety at Albert Einstein Healthcare Network in Philadelphia, PA. He is experienced in the use of behavior change processes in efforts to prevent medical errors and reduce health care-associated infections.